Managing Change in Primary Care

MIKE PRINGLE
JAS BILKHU
MIKE DORNAN
STEVE HEAD

with

PAULINE McAVOY
ROGER PRICE

and a foreword by
MARSHALL MARINKER

Illustrations by Bernard Cookson

RADCLIFFE MEDICAL PRESS
OXFORD

British Library Cataloguing in Publication Data

Making change in primary care.
1. Primary health services
I. Pringle, Mike

ISBN 1 870905 91 1

Typeset by Advance Typesetting Ltd, Oxford
Printed and bound in Great Britain

Contents

Foreword

SOME five years ago the authors of this book were brought together as a small group on one of the MSD Foundation's leadership courses for general practitioners. In the years subsequent to that course they continued to meet, and this book is one of the products of their work. It is a testament not only to their own enthusiasm and serious concern, but also to the intense spirit of professionalism in contemporary general practice.

What faces general practice in the coming decade is not simply the management of accelerating change whose pace we may predict with some certainty, but whose direction and content we can only wildly surmise. At the time of writing, general practice is coming to grips with a new contract whose construction and implementation will long furnish the most perfect example of how not to manage change.

The timing of this book, therefore, could not be more opportune. It is rooted not in management theory or social psychology, but in the actual experience of living in general practice partnerships, and of dealing with the day-to-day problems of management. The authors have recognized how imperative it will be for general practitioners (GPs) to master the diversity of skills and the work-load which general practice demands. They must do so if doctors and their colleagues are to make change happen, and not simply to react to the changes imposed by others.

I share with the authors a vision of the scope and importance of future general practice within a developing National Health Service (NHS). However, this vision of the future must belong not to a few enthusiastic protagonists, but to the vast majority of those who work in general practice. Unless general practitioners and their many co-workers in general practice develop a well-founded sense of ownership of the changes which will be brought about, there may be change, but there will not be real progress.

This book, with its practical orientation, its direct language and its lightness of touch, will I hope help many general practices to survive the first body blows of accelerating change, and then to begin the work of transforming their practices in accordance with their own professional values. It is too rarely stated that one of the key aims of good management in general practice should be the enhancement the quality of the professional lives of those who work in it.

As the person responsible for bringing this group of authors together, I am proud of their achievement and feel privileged to have been asked to introduce their work to the reader.

MARSHALL MARINKER
Director, MSD Foundation

Managing Change in Primary Care

Contributors

JAS BILKHU, *General Practitioner, Radcliffe-on-Trent, Nottinghamshire*

MIKE DORNAN, *General Practitioner, Chesterfield, Derbyshire*

STEPHEN HEAD, *General Practitioner, Ollerton, Nottinghamshire*

PAULINE MCAVOY, *General Practitioner, Auckland, New Zealand*

ROGER PRICE, *General Practitioner, Loughborough, Leicestershire*

MIKE PRINGLE, *Senior Lecturer, Department of General Practice, Nottingham and General Practitioner at Collingham, Nottinghamshire*

The Business Side of General Practice

Editorial Board

Preface

IT is a popular misconception, especially among politicians that general practices are unwilling to accept change. If you consider the changes of the past 20 years – in premises, staffing, record keeping, clinical standards, audit, vocational training – this seems an unlikely charge. But there are those who wish to force the pace of change.

Some practices seem to manage the changes they attempt better than others. Some practices seem to thrive on the oxygen of innovation, whilst others change little and late. Some practices have clear management structures, whilst others muddle through.

This book is constructed on the assumption that there are skills and techniques that can make the difference between these practices. Of course, nothing can overcome a truly destructive partnership, just as counselling cannot save a doomed marriage. But assuming that there is some potential in the situation, this book aims to identify the skills required to maximize the opportunities for change.

The origin of this book

The authors met as a group on an MSD leadership course in the Trent Region in 1983. We continued to meet regularly afterwards in order to provide each other with mutual support in personal and professional development. It quickly became apparent that this involved the identification of skills and techniques which were valuable in successfully managing change. These form the basis of this book.

The purpose of this book

By reading this book, you will increase your knowledge of the steps to be taken in managing change. We hope that you will achieve the following.

● You will increase your understanding of the personal and inter-personal aspects of the management of change.
● You will appreciate the benefits of managing change actively.
● You will be able to use material from the book to learn and practise the skills for the management of change and to untangle problems that arise in the practice.

We intend that parts of this book, especially the case studies and exercises, will be of use to vocational trainers, undergraduate teachers and organizers of courses for practice staff and doctors. Many of the principles are, however, general ones and this book may be of value to health service managers and other health professionals.

The content of this book

In writing this book we have set out to place the skills for the management of change in the context of our own experiences as active young general practitioners. These take the form of case studies of **true events** subtley altered to disguise the practice concerned which augment a descriptive text. Each section is accompanied by exercises which illustrate the issues raised in the text, whilst providing an opportunity to practise the skills required.

As you go through the book, you may recognize a problem from your own practice. We suggest that to gain insight you use a relevant exercise with other members of your primary health care team.

MIKE PRINGLE
April 1991

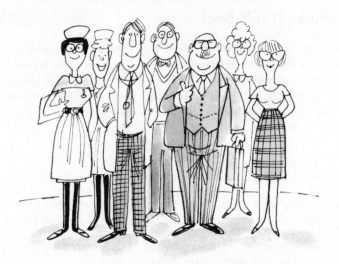

1 Introduction to the Management of Change

Contents of this chapter

Introduction

A degree in medicine is a wondrous thing. It appears to confer a right to patients' inner secrets and a profound knowledge of life; an ability to relate to people and handle the most difficult situations; teaching skills and a role in the community; but most alarming of all, a medical degree confers an ability to manage.

How this comes about is unclear – certainly management is poorly taught, except perhaps by example. However, at 28 a young doctor may find himself helping to manage a practice with 10,000 patients, four other partners (all idiosyncratic!), 15 or more staff, and a turnover of £250,000.

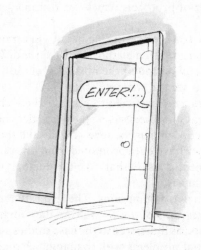

Often such a practice appoints a 'practice manager' who is usually an administrator with no management background and who is given no real training. The doctors and practice manager feel their way forward, the blind leading the blind, sometimes planning ahead but more usually reacting to changes once they become inevitable.

The pace of change can be phenomenal. One group member's practice, for example, has experienced the following changes in the past 12 years:

1 *Partnership.* Only one 'original partner' is still present out of a total of four. Twelve years ago the first vocationally trained partner joined the practice. Now three out of four are vocationally trained.
2 *Staff.* From a staff of a couple of receptionists there are now a practice manager, secretary, two practice nurses, and eight receptionists.
3 *Premises.* The practice has moved from the back of the senior partner's house where there were two small consulting rooms which were not sound-proof, to a new purpose-built health centre, which was owned by the District Health Authority (DHA) and is now owned by the practice under the cost rent scheme.
4 *Equipment.* Starting with an ancient ECG machine and a microscope the practice now has computers, nebulizers, tonometers, sterilizers, a defibrillator and a sonic aid.
5 *Services.* From offering a solely reactive service – responding only to patient demand – the practice has developed its prevention programme until it has become an integral part of everyday work. There is a successful patient participation group.
6 *Teaching.* The practice now has two vocational trainers and has a steady stream of medical students.
7 *Clinical.* The practice has had a formulary for nine years and has recently introduced a number of protocols which are routinely audited.

Any practice – indeed anybody working in any corner of primary care – could produce a similar list. After a plethora of Green and White Papers, new contracts and circulars, all on top of the normal evolution of primary care, we cannot consider that we are standing still.

However, the doctors were expected to manage these changes largely by instinct – in the best ways for themselves, their practices and their patients. In the last decade, practice managers have arrived like the cavalry. Unfortunately all too often they have been promoted from 'the ranks' and given no real training. Management is a skill that, like the doctors, they are expected to have acquired by osmosis.

This book is based on two assumptions. The first is that most practices do not manage the changes that occur as well as they might. Certainly the experience of the authors, as illustrated in the case studies, suggests that their practices have substantial problems with managing change.

The second assumption is that change can be managed effectively and that the techniques can be learnt. Not every attempt will succeed, but an awareness of the process of change and the techniques for managing it can increase the chances of success. Throughout the text there are case studies which are true examples from the practice lives of the authors. This case study illustrates the use of management of change techniques to achieve success.

CASE STUDY 1

Many ambitious GPs seek outside commitments, especially in vocational training schemes. For example one GP planned to apply for a course organizer post. The local scheme was facing disapproval. The trainers, none of whom were young, had become complacent, their practices often failed the regional criteria and trainers' workshops were poorly attended.

He applied for and was appointed to the post. He formed an agreement with the other, long-standing course organizer as to the division of labour and generally they agreed on both the problems (where are you now?) and the necessary solutions (where are you going?). His strategy rested mainly on setting up a group of young trainers for the future, who could compete for places on the scheme (how are you going to get there?). This stimulated the interest of some of the existing trainers and precipitated the departure of others. He made the half day release less didactic and improved the quality of the trainers' workshops.

This resulted in a substantial improvement in the scheme with tangibly improved morale; the scheme was visited and re-approved (how do you know when you have got there?) and the group member has become a well respected local course organizer.

Discussion points

1 This case study illustrates the various parts of the management of change process, this time successfully applied.
2 The GP worked with people, not against them; in particular he helped them to be involved in the changes as if they were their own initiatives.
3 Although this case study is outside the practice, it could just as easily have been a new partner joining a practice.
4 One problem for doctors in primary care is the absence of a career structure through which to enhance self-esteem and reputation. Outside activities therefore offer new challenges.

If this case study sounds too good to be true, it is one of the few where the GP met with unqualified success; but it serves to illustrate that change can come about in a predictable manner with a satisfactory outcome.

In this chapter the basic philosophy of managing change is explained and it is enlarged on in the subsequent chapters.

Principles in the management of change

Put simply, managing change is an exercise in navigation. You start with three simple questions:

- Where are you now?
- Where do you want to get to?
- How are you going to get there?

To these rather trite questions must be added a catalogue of second level ones:

- What were your experiences in getting to where you are?
- What are your overall aims and priorities?
- How does where you want to get to in this area fit in with your overall aims and priorities?
- What are the factors that help you and what factors will hinder you?
- What are the implications of different routes in getting to where you want to be?
- How will you know when you have arrived, or if you fail to arrive?
- How will you stop yourself when you get there and prevent your momentum from carrying you off course?

These questions highlight some of the issues in managing change. They are investigated further below.

Where are you now?

In order to set out on the road of change, a primary care team, like any team, needs to understand from where it starts. This includes the history of the practice, experience with similar changes and with change in general, and the roles of practice members in these changes.

Next it is important to know what motivates you and others around you. If you do not present the change as being compatible with the motivation of co-workers they will resist it.

Lastly you need to analyse carefully the problem itself, seeing it from your own viewpoint and that of others. You need to achieve a common perception of the problem among the members of the team, even if their individual reasons for wanting to address it differ.

Where do you want to get to?

Most problems have a solution, sometimes many of them. The art is to select the best one for the circumstances. For this you must look at the range of solutions and compare them with the goals of the practice and the goals of individual members of the practice.

The solution must then be 'sold'. This may involve persuading a key figure in the practice that they thought of or are personally responsible for putting forward this solution − the sharing of ownership of the idea.

Once there is common agreement on the change sought, the practice needs to decide on the method for achieving that change. In doing so it will define precisely the change desired, and thereby how to recognize when it has been achieved, or not as the case may be.

How do you get to where you want to be?

Actually managing the change when it is occurring is an art in itself. There are factors which will obstruct the change − obstructing factors − which need to be identified along with the helping factors. Resources need to be mobilized and the co-operation of all involved needs to be sought and maintained.

However, that is not all. The biggest problems with managing the process of change occur because responsibilities are not clear. The person who has the job of looking after the change has a mandate − and the quality of that mandate is a crucial determinant of the success of the process. [We apologize if the word 'mandate' appears to be jargon, but there is no suitable substitute. It means a commission by which a person or group requests another to act for them.]

Lines of accountability have to be established clearly, and this requires a level of formal organization in the decision making process of the team. The chairmanship and minutes of practice meetings and the control of delegation are important elements, as is the monitoring of the change as it is introduced.

How do you know when you have got there?

Change can get out of hand. Once the target has been reached, the situation needs to be reviewed. If further change is then necessary, so be it. If the situation is satisfactory, then let the change settle in for a while.

This book goes through these areas in turn, looking at the skills and the problems, and illustrating the text with real case studies. It finishes with an examination of the role of the practice manager in the new emerging primary care.

Of course the principles are not unique to primary care and can be applied in any walk of life. It is just that the need for these skills is particularly apparent in primary care and is likely to increase.

Learning points from Chapter 1

○ Change is all around you in primary care, and you often do not appreciate its extent or pace.
○ If change is managed, success is not guaranteed, but the chance of success is increased.
○ The management of change is a process with clearly definable steps, each with its skills and techniques.

2 Defining the Situation – Where Are You Now?

Contents of this chapter

Examining personal positions
Learning from the past
Defining the problem – for yourself and for others
Learning points

Introduction

The joke is told of the man who, on being asked the way to a distant town, replied 'Well, if I was you I wouldn't be starting from here'? Regrettably we too, usually set out from a less than ideal starting point in our journey of change. The art lies in accepting this fact and then using the initial position to its best advantage.

There is no clean slate. Even a doctor starting a practice from scratch has to accept the local population and social circumstances, the available staff and the contract with the Family Health Services Authority (FHSA). A practice manager in a busy practice may have five or more general practitioners, as many attached DHA nursing staff, a practice secretary, a couple of practice nurses and senior receptionists, not to mention a family and the world outside the practice to contend with.

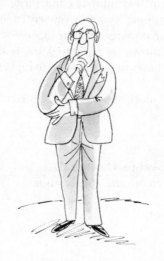

The more accurately you understand the current situation, the more effectively you will be able to plan, instigate and control change. The more you study it, the more complex the current position will become. You will need to identify the factors which will obstruct and aid change and take them into account.

If the process of change goes wrong, you should return to your assessment of the current situation. It might be that you have misjudged a person or a factor, or that you underestimated its effect on your plans.

Examining personal positions

You need to understand what motivates you and what your priorities are. This may seem superfluous. Surely you are not the problem, it is the others! This may be true, but you will benefit if you clarify your position.

Firstly you will be more prepared for the process of target setting. Secondly you will gain insights into what motivates and what the problems are of those around you. The factors that you will need to examine, for yourself and then for those around you, include:

● Motives and priorities
● Time allocation
● Talents

Motives and priorities

In choosing which changes to pursue and in planning those changes, you need to be sure of your own motives and those of others. What are your prime needs? If, for example, you are primarily concerned with your financial position, any change that increases your income will be attractive to you. If you are eager to be known as an innovator, both inside and outside the practice, then you are likely to be attracted to higher risk, perhaps expensive, options.

The factors which motivate you and your colleagues are likely to be included in this list:

● Physical achievement
● Stability (financial and psychological)
● Relationships and emotional appreciation
● Self-image
● Status and reputation
● Creativity

Exercise 1

Throughout the text of this book you will find a series of exercises. You will, of course, look at this one and decide that it has been put in for all those other readers! *We urge you to resist this temptation.*

None of the exercises is difficult. None requires hours of time. But you can use them to *understand* the ideas in the text in a way that you cannot by just reading this book.

For exercise 1, examine the list of motives (*see* page 8) and reflect on their relative importance in your life at the moment.

Then give each one a score (1 = low priority for you, 10 = high priority for you).

Ask someone you know and trust, for example a spouse, to rank these motives in relation to you. Others do not necessarily see us as we see ourselves – this has implications for when you assess your colleagues.

Take yourself back a decade. Try to remember what you were doing and to recall your aspirations. For each of the motives score and order them according to how you remember them to be ten years ago. Notice how motives change.

It is important to recognize the evolution of motives. As a generalization, children value stabililty, adolescents emphasize physical achievement and self-image, young adults work on relationships, and older adults look for recognition. Creativity is valued by all groups in selected individuals, but is often regarded with a degree of suspicion.

This evolutionary trail is, of course, highly simplistic and cannot be used judgmentally. If you jog daily and play squash twice a week, that does not infer that you are adolescent! However, it is useful to realize that motives often change with time.

Equally it is beneficial to know and understand those who work in the practice, particularly if the process of change is not to be beset with unnecessary surprises and reactions which could have been predicted.

Just as you have your motives, priorities, time conflicts and talents, so do the other members of your team. If you all shared similar motives and priorities, then establishing the need for change would be relatively straight-forward.

Many practices fail to manage change because there is a fundamental mismatch between the motives and therefore the priorities of members of the team. A junior partner wants to invest in an ECG machine because he or she wants to be a good clinician (self-esteem) and to be seen to be up-to-date (recognition), whereas a senior partner nearing retirement worries that he or she will not be good at interpreting ECGs (which threatens his self-esteem) and is interested in saving for his or her retirement (threatening his security).

CASE STUDY 2

This GP had a regular educational commitment every Friday afternoon which caused no disruption to visits or surgery (which she returned for in the evening). It did however create problems when she was the on-call doctor. She therefore approached a partner to see if the partner would regularly cover her for these few hours when on call.

Although the partner agreed, later the GP discovered that he was very upset at being asked. This was 'protected time' when the partner caught up on his paperwork. When she discovered that her partner was upset she was herself upset and angry. She felt that it was little to ask, especially since the income from the educational activity was pooled.

On reflection and discussion with the group, she understood the situation better. She valued the educational work highly since it enhanced her self-image and recognition. For her partner the obligation to cover appeared to infer a lack of recognition, and it conflicted with an activity that he deemed highly necessary – all this resulted in reduced self-esteem.

The GP approached another partner and arranged a mutual swap – an arrangement under which both doctors had equal status and equally serviced their needs.

Discussion points:

1 Clash of motives and priorities. The partner did not value the education activity and the GP did not value the paperwork.
2 Respect for others includes respecting how they prioritize their time. This is an essential part of a functional relationship.
3 This case study also illustrates that complex trade-offs are involved in pursuing a personal agenda, and trade-offs usually work better than one-way deals.

Never forget that every practice team evolves. The opportunity to replace a team member arises surprisingly often – at least once a year in a medium-sized practice. A high turnover can be a sign of poor morale, and every new appointment carries risks; but, while we have to accept the team to which we belong, personnel changes represent additional opportunities.

Exercise 2

List five major changes in your practice over the past two years. These will include those that you instituted, those that others espoused, some that are still underway, and others that were imposed from outside. They should all have involved you as a major player.

Consider the five changes carefully. Then characterize each change on a scale 'highly undesirable' (1) to 'highly desirable' (10) for you personally, and similarly on a scale of 1 to 10 for desirability for your organization (i.e. your practice).

Reflect carefully on how each of these changes relates to the motives of those in the practice and gain insight into how attitudes to changes are strongly influenced by motives.

CASE STUDY 3

Apparently out of the blue, a partner tendered his resignation from the partnership. He cited his need to return to his roots before his children were too old, and the need to offer a more personal level of care which was, he felt, not possible in a partnership.

The other partners felt upset and let down, but only one felt able to discuss the reasons for his resignation with the leaving partner. It transpired that there were more deep-seated problems. The leaving partner perceived there to be a lack of consistency both clinically and attitudinally in the partnership, and a lack of innovation.

The partners decided that, while they must appoint a new partner with whom they felt at ease, they should try to appoint somebody with innovative ideas.

Discussion points:

1 The disclosure of feelings and perceptions. You only find out what people really feel if you ask and listen.
2 How crises reveal underlying truths. It is all too easy to get so involved in coping with the crisis that the underlying problems are overlooked.
3 How crises may create attitudes and solutions which would have avoided the crisis to begin with.

Time allocation

The sensation of time pressure is a common experience. You all face demands on your time of varying importance from different sources. Sometimes you take on time consuming tasks and instantly regret it, but find it impossible to withdraw. As often as not time allocates itself, as if it were far beyond your control.

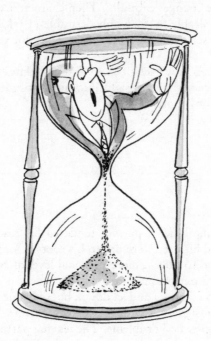

Indeed some time allocations may be beyond your control. Time spent sleeping can be rationed, but only up to a certain level. To continue to be employed it is necessary to attend work, to see patients. More of your time is under your control, however, than you think.

Doctors can, and do, change their appointment intervals and in the process dramatically alter their time allocations. Home visiting patterns vary widely from doctor to doctor. Medico-political involvement can be virtually half-time or nothing. Practice managers can get involved in reception desk cover, or can ensure staffing rotas to avoid it. They can get absorbed in the day to day running of the practice computer or they can delegate it.

The key lies in two areas: how you define your jobs and how you deal with competing pressures on your time.

Exercise 3

Draw a pie-chart (a circle that is partitioned like a cake, each slice representing a relative quality of time) that shows your current time allocation. Then draw another pie-chart to show the ideal time allocation for which you might realistically wish. The example shown here is for a theoretical GP (who obviously craves a quiet life without patients!). Please do not base your own charts on this one – think carefully about your time tasks and create charts that match your reality.

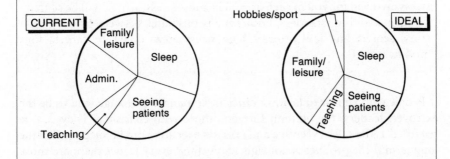

Ask the person identified for Exercise 1 to construct a pie-chart for your current time allocation and another for the ideal for your time allocation in their eyes. Compare your charts.

Your notion of what you feel your job to be is based on your explicit job description as might be generated before an interview, the understanding of your job held by others (including patients), your personal motives and the priorities and problems as you see them.

Competing time pressures can be coped with by accepting all tasks and failing in some (or even all) of them, accepting tasks up to a threshold of pressure, or by selecting out and accepting only those tasks that are 'high priority'. Such priority is judged by matching the tasks against your personal priorities.

Talents

Some people appear more influential than others – people listen to them, they get their way more than other people. This relates to the nebulous area of leadership. Everyone is a leader and a follower depending on the hierarchy of the group in which you find yourselves.

Exercise 4

Score each of the time slices on both your present and ideal pie-charts according to their time allocation priority, giving 1 to the highest priority and avoiding equal scores. For example, if socializing often eats into sleeping time, socializing will be given a lower score (higher priority) than sleeping. Examine the differences in priority between the present and the ideal − progress towards the ideal will be reflected in your personal aims.

Score each of the time slices on your present pie-chart according to the stress involved for you in each area. The most stressful area will be scored 1. Again avoid equal scores. Look for any mismatch between priority and stress scores: any low priority/high stress areas might be targets for modification.

People who appear to be most efficient at managing change tend to be the extrovert leaders, the opinion formers, those with charisma. They can be regarded as the sales executive and no sales executive can be successful in the long term if the product is not right. So behind every leader there are those who refine the product (the change that is to occur) and those who implement the changes which are agreed. At varying times you can play all three roles (generating ideas, selling them or sustaining them) − occasionally all at the same time − but your talents may lie more in one direction than another. There is nothing superior about any of these roles since each is an essential part of the process of change.

There are three other roles. There is the consumer of the change, who accepts it and will even support it in a passive way, but who relies on others to be the prime movers. Secondly, there is the person who obstructs change, overtly or covertly, actively or passively, because the changes clash with their priorities. The third role is assumed by the person who ignores the change. It seems peripheral to their priorities, too distant to be of concern. This can occur when the change is too small (it is delegated) or too distant ('there's nothing I can do').

So there are six identifiable roles which can be played in change:

- Generating ideas for change
- Selling ideas for change
- Sustaining the change
- Consuming the change
- Obstructing the change
- Ignoring the change

The first three roles all embody a personal commitment to the change, a concept which is called 'ownership' and which will be discussed later. The last three roles are essentially negative and infer no ownership of the change concerned.

A successful team needs members who have a range of talents for the first three roles. A team of totally like minds can be a recipe for stagnation. While virtually every change has passive consumers, all team members should be involved in the active roles for some changes while passively consuming others. Those who are always left to be passive consumers, quickly turn into obstructors or ignorers. So a successful team is one that has a variety of strengths which are exploited to the full.

Exercise 5

Consider these six roles in change. Take each of them and score each according to the extent to which you believe you have a talent for it. Score on a scale of 0 for no talent to 5 for a lot of talent.

Take the recent changes identified in Exercise 2. Identify for each change the role that most closely corresponds to your personal role.

Consider the similarities and differences between your talents and your roles.

Learning from the past

'We've tried that before and it didn't work'; 'we're not that sort of practice'. These familiar statements put forward as blocking manoeuvres may reflect current attitudes more than history, but the past can certainly colour the present. An understanding of that past can help explain current problems.

Further, a knowledge of the history, especially the times when changes went awry, can help you to anticipate and avoid problems with your changes. History does not just involve facts, although establishing these is the first step. It crucially involves the interpretation of behaviour. Why didn't the practice favour a move to new premises when it was last discussed? What happened when one partner tried to introduce a diabetic mini-clinic five years ago?

The best, but most biased, sources of answers are the older workers in the practice – the partners, the senior receptionists and the longer term attached staff; minutes of practice meetings and correspondence can help. One of the most important guides is how people feel now. When discussing distant events (which should now be safe), watch carefully how they respond to your enquiries.

If you are proposing a change similar to one that you know to have failed before, prepare the ground carefully. Be prepared to present your change as quite different from the previous failure, to explain why this one might succeed where the other failed and to accept the feelings that might be aroused by memories of a previous fiasco. To ignore the past is to court failure.

CASE STUDY 4

This issue of learning from the past is emphasized by another case report. A GP wanted to introduce chronic disease protocols into his practice, but he was not keen to do all the work himself. He raised the possibility of a diabetes protocol at a practice meeting and this was taken up by the trainee.

The trainee was slow to produce a first draft and when it was produced it was clearly inadequate. At the trainee's request the trainer became involved and after another long wait the ensuing protocol was greeted with open disagreement. The partners could not agree screening intervals, nor the content of screening. Discussion got bogged down on the role of the nurse and of separate diabetic mini-clinics. The protocol was shelved.

Several months later a local initiative was started whereby diabetic patients could be referred to opticians for regular fundoscopy. This reopened the protocol issue, but previous experience was a major deterrent to progress.

In the discussion it became clear that the previous initiative had been poorly organized and the delegation to the trainee had been inadequately supervised. Furthermore, all the doctors expressed high levels of anxiety over the adequacy of their fundoscopy, something which had not been openly discussed on the previous occasion.

Since these problems had now been removed the protocol was resurrected, and was implemented within a few weeks. Immediately activity began on an array of other protocols – the log jam had been broken.

Discussion points:

1 The importance of trying to understand the underlying problems and the real reasons for past failure.
2 Inappropriate delegation and its long term effects.

Defining the problems – for yourself and for others

As part of any consideration of the current situation, you must define your major problems. Although this overlaps with target-setting, some problems are not amenable to a cure and may not feature in a realistic list of targets.

In reading this chapter, and in doing the exercises, your problems should have become evident and you should be in a position to place them under a number of headings:

1 Structure (e.g. premises, practice area/size)
2 Personnel
3 Time
4 Finance
5 Expectations (internal and external)
6 Imposed changes

Of these only the last two need explanation. An imposed change is one that is inevitable and over which you and your colleagues have no direct influence. In companies (and health authorities) it is commonplace – a memorandum from the managing director, a new strategy from the board, a take-over. In general practice it mainly consists of contractural changes or unilateral decisions by the DHA. Coping with imposed change is discussed later.

Exercise 6

Draw up a list of the major problems facing your practice under each of the above headings (structure, personnel etc).

Consider what other key co-workers (partners, manager etc) might think are the major problems that you face. Approach a co-worker whom you trust and ask them to draw up a similar list of major problems facing the practice. Compare the results.

Expectations can be internal, i.e. they relate to your own personal expectations and to those of the organization itself. The practice might view itself as highly efficient, or very approachable, or particularly caring. Expectations can also be external, i.e. those of the government and patients.

If there is a common perception of these problems then the practice is very fortunate. It is, however, unlikely that this is the case, and it is helpful therefore to understand the different perceptions that surround you. This may be clear to you already, but asking co-workers for their list of problems may reveal surprises.

CASE STUDY 5

Dr W reported on an initial near disaster but final success in his practice which had identified a need for, and obtained official approval for, a new partner. It was initially agreed that this new partner should be female. However the best applicants were all male and these were whittled down to a final two.

At the practice meeting to make the final choice one partner was particularly silent. One applicant had won the approval of the other partners and was approved as the candidate of choice, but fortunately the partners gave themselves two days to sleep on the decision before acting.

In the intervening perod the silent partner's feelings came to the surface. He felt that the need to appoint a partner and the hard logic of the choice was overriding his gut feelings about the candidate and the previously stated need for a female partner.

In further discussions it was clear that the practice had hardly discussed its preferences for the new partner and how best to obtain the ideal person. Therefore, the advertisement and partnership description might have put female applicants off. Also the need for a new partner to cope with increasing workload had become the perceived priority, and so the appointment process had been like a steam-roller.

After more detailed discussions of the precise problems and needs of the practice, they decided to re-advertise, making the job more accessible to female doctors, and received some high quality applications from women.

Discussion points:

1 The problem was originally defined as 'we need a female partner' but this got lost, and the selection process went astray.
2 The need to make the problems, needs and priorities of the practice explicit through discussion. (Beware the silent person).
3 Partnership changes are particularly fraught, since selection results can dramatically influence the future.
4 There is a spectrum of behaviour varying from the completely logical to the intuitive (but inexplicable). Both ends of the spectrum have their place.

Learning points from Chapter 2

○ It is necessary to understand your own personal motives and those of colleagues.
○ Events in the past can heavily influence attitudes to proposals – the past needs to be accepted and overcome.
○ A clear shared analysis of problems and priorities is the basis on which to make sound decisions for the mangement of change.

Setting Sights – Where Are You Going?

Contents of this chapter

Setting personal goals
Revealing the goals of others
Seeking a consensus on goals
Ownership of ideas
Defining the change sought (overall and intermediate aims)
Selecting the strategy for the process of change
Defining the criteria for success and failure
Defining time-scale
Learning points

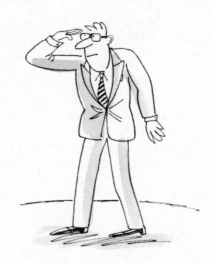

Introduction

In the first chapter of this book the question was 'where am I?' In this chapter the next logical question is addressed: 'where do I want to be?' There is little merit in change for change's sake, so a direction for change is necessary. However, simply setting out in a general direction can be fruitless if you have no firm idea of the distance to travel and how to recognize that you have arrived.

This may sound pedantic. If, for example, a practice perceives a need for a practice nurse, then surely it is clear cut – the change has succeeded when a nurse is in post. Suppose the problem that precipitated her appointment was a low cervical cytology uptake, and the nurse is not trained to take cervical smears? Suppose even that you did not have a low cervical smear rate, you just thought you did? Has the outcome been successful?

Before instituting any change it is necessary to define the problem and to identify a solution to that problem, which does not create in its wake greater problems than the one being solved. Only then can you define how you will judge whether the change has been successful. Then you can begin to put the change into place.

For small changes much of this can be implicit. For anything significant, the processes must be explicit if substantial risks are to be avoided.

Setting personal goals

Managing change is about managing yourself first.

Much of your education has been about observing and understanding other people and things: however, to do this effectively requires a firm 'home base' in self-awareness and self-management.

The first task is to define your personal goals. This may sound similar to defining your motives, but it is in fact quite different. Knowing what drives you is one thing – knowing where you want to be driven is quite another. Time and energies are limited, and loyalties are often conflicting. Your personal goals need to take account of this, in an honest and realistic manner. Personal goals must be personal: in confidence to yourself or to those very close (e.g. a spouse). There are many reasons for this including false modesty and fear of failure.

Personal goals need to be considered over differing time-scales: for practical purposes, short, medium and long term are useful concepts. Goals can also be divided according to which part of life they relate to. Conventionally three areas can be recognized: self, family and work, with the latter divided into work (i.e. the practice) and other professional activities (i.e. activities outside the practice).

Exercise 7

Fill in this grid with your personal goals.

TIME-SCALE: SHORT   MEDIUM   LONG

Self

Family

Practice

Other professional

Fill in a similar grid, only entering those items that you think you will be able to share with your colleagues. All the items on this second grid should appear on the first, but there will be some items on the first which are too sensitive to share on the second grid.

Revealing the goals of others

Failure to recognize differences in goals between members of the practice can lead to persistent unhappy and frustrating work situations.

CASE STUDY 6

Disparities in workload are a common cause of partnership tension. This is illustrated by Dr F who tells of resentments that had built up in his practice. The partners booked surgeries of equal lengths but had different appointment durations. This meant that some partners saw more patients. Also those with the shorter appointments tended to finish first and therefore see more urgent end-of-surgery cases.

This problem overflowed into outside appointments. One of the high workload doctors was a course organizer and resented pooling her income when she got no workload relief. Another high workload partner resisted becoming a trainer because he knew the other partners would not allow a compensatory adjustment in patient load.

In discussions it became clear that this workload problem was the tip of the iceberg. The partners did not relate well to each other (although they did profess to like each other) and they had very different goals. While completing consultations was a shared goal, it was not being achieved equally; teaching and external activities were non-shared goals.

Discussion points:

1 The problems of long-standing resentments arising from incompatible goals.
2 The benefits of open discussion.
3 Additionally, although no obvious solution had been found, understanding was increased, making future co-operation more likely. In fact the problem was resolved several years later.

To manage change requires an awareness of what others involved think and feel. In addition, it is necessary to understand the goals of others. Just as your goals are often personal, and therefore difficult to share, so the goals of others may be deliberately withheld from you.

To reveal those goals requires, therefore, a level of observation and interpretation that exceeds that commonly taken for granted in working relationships. Its achievement requires continual effort and awareness.

'Are you listening or waiting to speak?'

Talking and listening are essential skills in both medicine and management. Many of the principles of good general practice consulting (open-ended questions, non-directive counselling, empathy, reflection etc.) have the same relevance and validity when communicating with colleagues.

Assessing underlying motives, or what makes people tick, is in many ways analogous to the classical diagnostic process. Similarly, there are parallels between anticipatory care and the need to keep one step ahead in assessing others and predicting their future reactions.

It is, however, often difficult to transfer communication skills from the consultation situation to the management situation. This is usually due to two obvious differences – management tends to be done with people we know are already well informed; and the relationship is perceived as being more equal, adult, and therefore less indulgent.

CASE STUDY 7

As a course organizer, Dr H had been approached by a trainee who had various problems, none of which would on its own be significant. However, since the accumulation of problems indicated that something might be amiss, the GP decided to make an informal visit to the practice.

He prepared by considering all the possible ways in which he might handle the visit, all of which involved being 'active'. In the event he found himself listening as a major practice problem was revealed. The trainer talked himself into the conclusion that it would be best to resign and the course organizer was helpful in counselling the trainer on how best this might be managed.

Discussion points:

1 Pre-meeting preparation was useful, but turned out to be irrelevant.
2 The skills are those of a GP – history-taking, listening, empathizing, counselling and breaking bad news.

People sometimes fail to react to situations as you might expect. This may be because of unreasonable assumptions on your part, or a degree of mis-representation on the part of others – often it is a mixture of both. In a gush of enthusiasm it is easy to neglect the deeper, less overt feelings of others: equally people sometimes have difficulty, or are reluctant, to express their reservations openly.

The better your understanding of those you work with, the greater your chance of correctly assessing their motives and goals. However, in some areas the problem can be alleviated by making goal setting overt, especially in the work area. In addition, some structured thinking can reveal the most obvious of your colleagues' goals.

Exercise 8

Ask your key co-workers to reveal their work goals, by asking them to leap forward five years and to list the major changes that they would like to see in place by then. Ask them then to write beside each a year number (1 for this year, 4 for fourth year etc.) for when they think that change may occur. Do the same exercise yourself and arrange a meeting to discuss the answers.

Then, for each of your key co-workers, try to make a statement on themes that dominate their lives using the following headings, plus others you may wish to add:

Career	present status, prospects, perception of job
Life stage	age, marital and parental status, family commitments, personal health, energy, stamina
Pleasures	interests, hobbies, priorities, ambitions
Anxieties	pre-occupations, fears, perceived weaknesses
Values	political, religious and philosophical factors

If a change fails because people do not share your vision, or because they appear to agree with it and then obstruct it, re-assess your perception of the goals for each person concerned and the reason may become obvious. Equally, it may be helpful to precede the first mention of a tricky change with a re-examination of goals.

Seeking a consensus on goals

When everybody in an organization shares the same goals, matters are greatly simplified – it only remains to decide how and at what pace each goal is to be achieve. This is, unfortunately, seldom the case. It is necessary therefore to identify those goals that are shared and those that might become shared with increased understanding.

Other goals might be traded. For example, if one partner in a practice is very keen to set up a diabetic clinic, the others may react with indifference or concern that this will use too much nurse time. By identifying that one partner is keen to be a trainer and another wishes to reorganize the appointments system, the partner wanting the diabetic clinic can trade his or her support. This is, in effect, what often happens – awareness of the process increases the chances that it will be managed successfully.

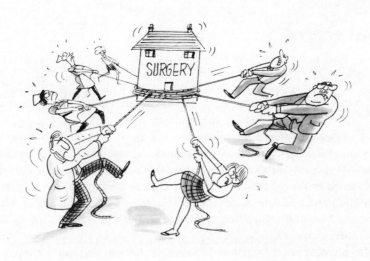

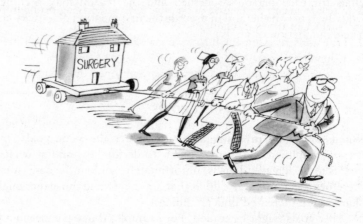

In this process of seeking consensus, thought must be given to those who appear relatively neutral and undemanding. Unspoken frustrations can simmer and have a more disruptive effect on the management process than overtly expressed antagonism.

CASE STUDY 8

Problems with 'silent partners' and poor decision making surfaces in this case study. A partner in Dr B's practice had become increasingly involved with a hospital appointment which, while bringing in a good income, was causing problems with work-load in the practice.

This partner offered the solution of taking on a women's retainer scheme doctor and, it transpired, knew a suitable candidate. At the meeting to discuss this proposal one partner was particularly quiet. At the interview the woman was offered the job without a chance for the partners to discuss the appointment, and afterwards the silent partner exploded in anger. He felt he had not been fully consulted and that the work in the practice should take precedence over outside work.

Dr B called another meeting to discuss these underlying feelings. After a full discussion it was agreed to continue with the appointment and for the partner to continue the outside work. However the dissenting partner felt that his views had been valued.

Discussion points:

1 Work-load can be a cause of friction with underlying problems coming to the surface in times of change.
2 True consensus means informed consensus in which each member feels that they have contributed.
3 Confronting problems as they arise with open discussion.

When presenting ideas and seeking a consensus you will need to use the following skills. To be able to:

- Seek opinions and feelings beforehand
- Emphasize areas of common interest
- Provide attractive offers for others
- Plan for trade-offs
- Maintain a sound negotiating stance
- Bear in mind the anxieties of others
- Present a package which people cannot refuse
- Acknowledge drawbacks honestly
- Allow time for the discussion
- Allow time for a consensus to develop
- Back off and re-think rather than force a losing issue

Never forget that success is most likely if the change solves a problem for all the participants. The less this is the case the more difficult consensus is to achieve.

Exercise 9

Revisit Exercise 2 (page 11) where you constructed a list of recent changes in your practice.

Identify for each one how a consensus was reached, and in particular what led you to agree to each one. Identify the process which led to its adoption, and in particular the skills used from the above list.

Ownership of ideas

The 'ownership of ideas' sounds like American jargon which is devoid of meaning. We have sought for a better way to express this idea, but this phrase seems to be the only one that suits. Every idea has to have at least one 'owner' if it is to be accepted, and usually the more owners the better.

As a rule, one person, or a small group of people, are perceived as having more ownership of an idea than others. Margaret Thatcher was, for example, identified as the owner of the poll tax, and Kenneth Clarke as the owner of the NHS reforms. In reality, the poll tax idea came from a think-tank and the NHS reforms were already rolling before Clarke returned to the Ministry of Health. It is not crucial, therefore, who thought up an idea; it is crucial that someone with authority is seen to own that idea and to be identified with it.

Where an idea has come from is usually assumed to be obvious, although the truth may be wildly different. There are many reasons why it is often useful and sometimes essential for the innovator or prime mover behind an idea to sacrifice ownership as a price for effective implementation, among them:

1 *Pride*. People and organizations often react badly to being presented with ideas which they feel they should have thought of first
2 *Fear of the unknown*. Common enough, but people or organizations tend to cope with innovation far better if they feel it *belongs* to them
3 *Competition*. For various reasons people are often competing against each other, maybe for status or promotion. To turn competition into co-operation often requires sharing ownership of the ideas

For these reasons, you may well find yourself passing on the ownership of some ideas to others in order to increase their chance of success. You may alternatively wish to retain prime ownership while spreading the ownership of smaller stakes around a number of other members of the practice team.

The ownership of ideas is to do with a feeling that you share in its ultimate fate. While one person or a group retains the first ownership, small stakes need to be given to those that take up the idea. When people are speaking for or voting for an idea, ownership is, in part, transferred.

If an idea is to be successfully implemented, those involved need to feel part of the idea. The acid test of ownership is – how would I feel if this idea failed? If you own a part of it, you care about its failure. If you do not own it, you will probably not mourn its passing.

Evidently the wider the ownership the better, and a consensus goal starts with mutual ownership. However selling the ownership may be difficult, and it is imperative that the stakes do not become so small that nobody cares enough to invest in making it work.

So how can you sell the ownership of ideas? There are some recognizable strategies:

● Seek and acknowledge views before formulating the idea
● Allow others to change the idea so that a part of it becomes theirs
● Seek help in presenting and carrying forward the idea
● Allow others to espouse the idea
● Resist the temptation to be possessive about ideas
● Share ideas and goals rather than solutions

A key decision is the extent to which the idea will continue to be identified with yourself. Sometimes it is best to surrender the trappings of ownership, while remaining vigilant in the shadows. In such proxy leadership another person is given the idea to present and develop.

Leading from behind is a high risk strategy, based on placing others in a position from which they will emerge with the conclusions you expect or want. It may however offer the best chance of success if your time is limited, or there are relationship or historical reasons why you are less likely to get the idea adopted. The snag with this yielding of ownership is that your own contribution and value may not be recognized, but this self-effacement may be the necessary price for success.

Being a chairman, although often equated with leadership, is a circumstance in which delegated ownership is often necessary. The chair can be a difficult position from which to innovate: ideas may well need delegation to be fed back up your particular organization. Conversely, sacrificing the role of chairman might be the most effective way to attain a position of power to advance new ideas.

CASE STUDY 9

Practice managers, in common with others in administrative positions in health care, often have a creditibility problem with clinical workers.

This case study illustrates the need to listen carefully. Before the 1990 Contract, the problem of new registrations was discussed in Dr T's practice and the suggestion was made that, on registering, they might be given a new patient questionnaire. When they returned it, the patient could be invited to an initial assessment interview with the practice nurse.

The practice manager argued against this, saying that new patients are too busy moving house to bother filling in forms. She suggested that it would be better to do it after three months.

However, the partners decided that it would be better to give out the questionnaires straight away, and the first 50 families to register were given questionnaires and appointments with the nurse. The acceptance rate was only 20%.

The practice then decided to do things the practice manager's way and this has now become the established practice.

Discussion points:

1 The need to canvass and listen to all views.
2 Be brave enough to back down if events prove you wrong.

3 The need for doctors and practice managers to pull together. Lack of enthusiasm or dissension by a partner or the practice manager is likely to be transmitted to the rest of the staff.
4 Audit the result of decisions, particularly if controversial.

Tact and delegated presentation may, regrettably, be essential tactics for non-clinical staff to have their ideas given the serious consideration they deserve.

Ideas in general practice often come from people who are not full-time staff. This is hardly surprising since they have more opportunity to sample other ideas elsewhere. However when it comes to presentation this advantage of broader networking can be lost in the type of downgrading often experienced with ideas from non-clinicians, and part-time GPs.

Young principals can have similar experiences, often finding that good ideas they have brought from elsewhere cannot be effectively introduced by them alone.

In all these cases it may be necessary to sell overtly or covertly the majority ownership in an idea in order to further its chances of success. In most instances, however, it is only necessary to surrender minority interests, and this leaves you with the principal ownership, and responsibility.

Exercise 10

Consider the list of recent changes as drawn up in Exercise 2 and developed in Exercise 9.

If possible identify in each case who actually started the idea rolling (i.e. who had initial ownership), who later supported it and who is now seen as the main holder of the idea (i.e. who has shared in the ownership and whether the original owner has surrendered majority or minority shares in the idea).

Sometimes you present an idea but fail to gain acceptance of it. This may be because the idea is a poor one; or it may not meet the priorities of the practice; or it may need to be presented with different ownership. However, all may not be lost because the seed may be sown. The problem may just be one of timescale and the idea may have to develop and take root.

Getting the momentum for change going is sometimes the hardest part, and often the partnership may perceive other issues as having greater priority. If an idea is good it may well work its way into the culture of the practice until its adoption seems a natural progression. Initial rejection is, therefore, not necessarily a disaster – it might be the precursor to a wider ownership and sponsorship within the practice. So do not be surprised if ideas which you propose fail the first time, only to find a better time and a different owner later.

CASE STUDY 10

Four years previously Dr K had put forward the idea of employing a practice nurse specifically for prevention, to run the call and recall registers, to help with screening and immunizations and to keep the practice informed of its level of preventive activity through regular audits. The partners instead decided to opt for a clerical worker who would do the figures only.

As the practice expanded, the problem of new staffing came up again. At this meeting one of the other partners enthusiastically proposed a new idea – a practice nurse for prevention. This was supported by the partners and was implemented. The half-time post was filled with a very capable local nurse and proved so successful that a year later a full-time prevention nurse was recruited to further the work.

Discussion points:

1 Bide your time.
2 The ownership of the idea may change.
3 The initial change is often the hardest. Once the momentum is going, further change gets easier.

Defining the change sought (overall and intermediate aims)

Desired change must be carefully defined and the aim should be understood by all involved (unless deliberate decisions not to do this are made). Without clearly defined targets, misunderstandings are likely to arise over what the change is, how it can be achieved, and who does what in that process.

It is easy to miss the definition stage because it appears so self-evident, but it can be the root of many misunderstandings. Suppose that a practice agrees that a new initiative is required in disease prevention. Some partners may understand by this term opportunistic screening for hypertension, others well-person clinics, while others may think of vaccinations and immunizations. Unless everybody is thinking along the same lines, trouble is being stored up for a later stage.

It would be better, instead of gaining an ill-defined consensus, to put forward a set of aims, each of which is part of the change being sought. Some would be short/medium term, while others are longer term. Each partner can then consider each of the aims and voice hopes and fears concerning each. When consensus is reached (which might require surrendering some aims) it is an informed consensus which is much more likely to last.

The secret of defining the change is, whenever possible, to present it in writing and in a form that allows assessment of achievement later. The change illustrated above might be presented thus:

Overall aim	To improve the early detection of disease in this practice.
	Although primary prevention (immuniz- ation etc.) is important, this proposal is for improved early detection (secondary prevention).
Aims	To increase screening for hypertension in adults aged 35–70 years, so that a blood pressure measurement within the past five years is recorded in 90% of records.
	To increase the cervical cytology uptake to over 80% of those women aged 25–64 years who have not had a hysterectomy.
	To screen high risk groups for hyperlipid- aemia.

And so on. Obviously such a document needs to be accompanied by a proposition for achieving these aims, but at least the intended change is evident to all.

Selecting the strategy for the process of change

Selecting the strategy follows logically on from the statement of aims. Since the available strategies are legion, only general advice can be given here.

The basic principle is to enunciate clearly a strategy for achieving the change sought, then to return to the aims to check that this strategy can actually achieve them all. If it cannot, be explicit about that.

For example, if the problem is repeat prescribing, you may have a dozen subsidiary aims which range from checking compliance to running a drug ordering system for the dispensary. The strategy might be to buy a computer, and persuade the practice of the idea in principle. You then visit the computer suppliers, and find that those with the best clinical systems have the worst dispensary features and vice versa. You then need to present a choice to the practice in terms of the original aims, with or without a firm recommendation.

In addition to choosing a strategy and following the simplistic basic pathway, there are some other considerations:

Gradual or sudden changes

A change can be phased in over a period of time (permits modification as change progresses) or introduced on one predetermined day.

Rigid or vague description

A proposal can be rigidly described/predetermined or can be presented in vaguer form encouraging evolutionary improvement but risking reactive fudging.

Ambiguous or unambiguous presentation

Change can be presented in an unambiguous way (so that everybody knows where they stand), or more ambiguously (so that apparent consensus is easier but later retrospective disagreement more likely). The latter is only recommended if it has clearly worked with some key co-workers in the past.

High or low risk techniques

Techniques for implementation can be high or low risk: usually there is a correlation between risk and higher reward potential.

Overt and covert planning

Your planning can be overt or covert: clearly neither is ever possible absolutely, but how much do you tell, to whom and when? Overt planning can introduce the change to people gradually and prepare a consensus, but it can also alert the reactionaries. Only occasionally is the sudden revealing of a plan effective, and this is usually when a crisis occurs and solutions are urgently sought.

Defining the criteria for success or failure

You may feel that it is obvious whether an idea has succeeded or failed, but this is often not so. Success and failure are complex qualities with several aspects to each. When involved in difficult changes within already complex situations, a clear view of the end-point and a clear definition of successful or unsuccessful outcome are essential.

Criteria can be judged in terms of yourself, the practice and others. They can also be subdivided into major criteria and peripheral criteria. The design of criteria can affect your vulnerability: the more readily others can monitor the change, the more vulnerable you are. However, you should always be able to make an honest appraisal yourself.

If you have a good set of aims these can act as your success/failure criteria, but there may be other more subtle criteria to add. The introduction of a practice nurse might, for example, be a way of preparing the ground for a diabetic clinic. It would be unwise to make this explicit, but it could be a personal success criterion.

Defining time-scale

Change cannot be considered sensibly without linking it to a time-scale. There are many factors which determine this, including:

● The physical and financial situation
● The attitudes of those involved
● External factors such as imposed time-scales

Some aspects of time-scale are fixed, others are capable of change. If several parts of the process occur simultaneously, the overall rate of progress will be equal to (i.e. be limited by) the slowest part. If several parts have to occur consecutively and in order, then the minimum for achieving these will be the sum of all consecutive parts.

The essential lesson here is to consider critically the time-scale of any proposed change and make it as realistic as possible. If it is too short then failure is built into the change. If it is too long then momentum will be lost.

Exercise 11

Consider the 1989 White Paper *Working for Patients* in light of the comments in Chapter 2 of this book. Analyse the proposed changes, not in terms of the effect on yourself or your colleagues, but as an exercise in change. In particular consider how the following skills were and were not used:

● Seeking consensus on goals
● Ownership of ideas
● Defining the change sought
● Selection of strategy for the process of change
● Defining the criteria for success or failure
● Defining the time-scale

Consider how this proposal for change might have been better prepared.

Learning points from Chapter 3

○ Goals, especially the goals of others, must be carefully defined; as must the nature of desired change.
○ Success is most likely if it solves a problem for all participants.
○ Many skills used in clinical work are of value in managing others, especially in assessing other people's goals.
○ It is often useful and sometimes essential for the prime mover behind an idea to sacrifice ownership as the price of effective implementation.
○ Non-clinical and part-time workers in the practice often have much to offer but lower credibility in the promotion of change.
○ In order to assess progress, or lack of it, criteria for success must be defined.

4 Getting Change Started – How Are You Going to Get There? (Part One)

Contents of this chapter

Securing and defining a mandate with commitment
Clarifying current resources
Identifying obstructions and planning to avoid them
Identifying and mobilizing helping factors
Coping with imposed change
Learning points

Introduction

Having defined where you are and where you want to be, and having identified the route to get there, you must get the process of change underway. This sounds easy, but is often the hardest and most neglected part of the management of change.

Once a change has been presented and agreed, it develops a momentum all of its own. When everybody has agreed on the problem and the solution, the change will start almost by default. In looking back over failed changes, this is often the point when problems really started.

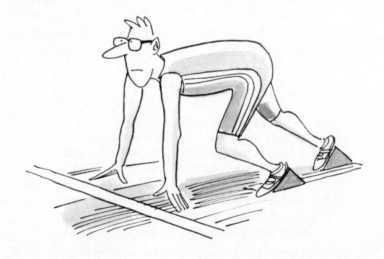

Change needs control. Change needs supervision. Change needs nurturing. Change needs monitoring.

In managing change while it takes place, special skills are required and these are discussed in this chapter. The most important skill lies in securing, defining and sustaining a mandate. This is an unattractive word, but it is, with the ownership of ideas, a piece of jargon that does not really have a substitute. Therefore, a prime task of this chapter is to define what we mean by a mandate and to describe a mandate's importance.

Securing and defining a mandate with commitment

THE MANDATE DEFINITION

Mission to accomplish
Acquired authority
Never abused
Delegated powers
Assigned task
Trust bestowed
Errand to accomplish

A mandate is the right by which a person acts in the name of another. It can be given or taken by individuals or groups. Examples of each are:

	Taken	Given
Individual	Dictator/senior partner	Practice manager for e.g. staff wages
Group	The government for matters not in manifesto	Manager and partner e.g. computerization

Taken mandates

Mandates are taken by people or groups in powerful positions. Their power derives from history, their personalities and an implicit authority. In primary care the classic example is a senior partner, but autocratic district managers and employers are other examples.

These mandates are high risk, and potentially high gain. They do not rest on an explicit consensus and often command very narrow ownership, so it is easy for those affected by the change involved to resent the mandate. By inhibiting constructive discussion, a taken mandate may rest on an incorrect assessment of the problem or its solution. Lastly, if mandates are taken in one area, this may inhibit people from seeking mandates in others, since they perceive the futility of doing so.

Those in a position to take mandates are also in a position to give them without consultation, and short of a revolution (confronting the senior partner and winning – which is the ultimate solution) the only way of coping is to be ready to seek a mandate when the opportunity arises. Even the most autocratic of partners has needs and these can be traded for mandates. They might, for example, wish you to do a surgery for them, and this can be linked to a mandate to examine the rota.

Proceeding without a mandate is equivalent to taking a mandate. It is high risk if you are not powerful enough to sustain it, and by putting yourself into the 'taken mandate' category you are risking all the resentment and negative reactions that this engenders.

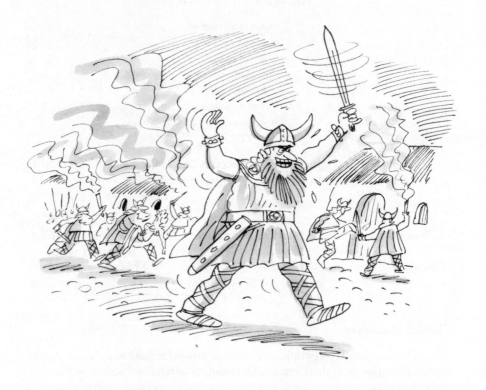

Given mandates

Mandates are given by a consensus of the whole group, or may be retained within the whole group. For example, a practice meeting might agree that it needs to consider a Patient Participation Group and could give a mandate to one member, or a group of members, to explore the area. It could, however, decide to have a special meeting of the whole group to consider it further, keeping the mandate within the group itself.

At the beginning of the process of change a mandate is often left deliberately vague. Somebody is asked to 'consider', 'explore' or 'look at' a problem. It is essential that such a mandate is not abused by moving into specific areas – a mandate to explore a Patient Participation Group is not a mandate to approach a possible chairman and arrange the first meeting; a mandate to be responsible for immunization does not include writing to other doctors' patients.

CASE STUDY 11

This case study presents a problem that has been created when a partner was given a mandate which was then exceeded.

Dr P's partnership had agreed that the practice's activities in preventive care needed to be improved. Simultaneously, for the first time, specific tasks were allocated to particular partners, so one partner was given the task of the 'executive role' for immunization and paediatric surveillance.

The problem arose because this partner perceived the task to include taking any action which he thought appropriate. Letters were sent to defaulting patients which were 'too threatening' for Dr P, although they would appear to patients to have been sent with his approval. At a meeting called to confront this issue, the partner given responsibility for preventive care failed to attend and the next day issued an ultimatum that the practice should back him or he would relinquish his role.

A compromise was finally reached whereby each partner should sign, and thus approve, any letter sent out to a family with which he was concerned.

Discussion points:

1 Clarity of mandates is important. Since the partnership had never delegated specific tasks before, it was not surprising that it failed to appreciate the need to specify the mandate in detail, including when to report back.
2 A mandate infers a democratic rather than autocratic right to act on behalf of others. The partner who confused the two found himself very exposed, which explains the disruptive effects of his behaviour.
3 Valuing the efforts of others; valuing the relationship between individual doctors and their patients.
4 Practice meetings. Holding formal meetings with minutes, decisions, 'action by' a named person and 'report back' at agreed intervals can help avoid these problems.

It is necessary to define the mandate. After an initial exploration, you need to report back to the whole group and seek a consensus on your aims and strategy. Then you are in a position to seek a defined mandate, although the group may choose to give such a mandate to somebody else. Whenever possible ensure that such a mandate is recorded in the minutes of the meeting. If this is an intermediate mandate, then return later to get the full mandate. Some mandates in complex changes are phased. You gain a mandate for the first stage, but the group retains the right to reconsider at the end of that stage before giving another mandate to continue.

Exceed your mandate at your peril. If in doubt, return to the main group to redefine or re-establish your mandate. If a mandate has been given, it can be withdrawn – if you sense that you have lost the consensus, go back a stage and try to regain the mandate or you risk having a taken mandate instead.

The essence of a good mandate is commitment. If all, not just most, of the main group are committed to the mandate given (rather than being browbeaten into it), they are much less likely to withdraw their support. The strongest mandate is one given by the group after a full discussion of written documentation, preferably on several occasions, and with the mandate recorded in the minutes.

Exercise 12

Consider again the list of recent changes drawn up in Exercise 2.

For each one record the type of mandate and its strength.

For those changes that you personally espoused, consider how you defined and achieved your mandate, and how much commitment your key co-workers gave to it.

You need to beware of the silent agreer to a decision or mandate who may in fact disagree, not understand or not wish to participate. These people tend to feel little or no involvement with the decision and therefore may sabotage progress at a later date with dire consequences. Case Study 5 is an example of this.

Once a mandate has been given to somebody in your group, leave it to them to get on with it while offering firm moral support (*see* Case Study 12). This does not exclude being directly involved when requested, but mandate holders need to be given the trust and space to carry out their mandate without tinkering or unnecessary interference.

CASE STUDY 12

The case study relates problems with action after decisions taken in practice meetings. Dr E's partnership had agreed to develop a protocol for hypertension so that the practice nurse could help with routine reviews and one partner had volunteered for the task. While most of the protocol was easy, she had, however, got bogged down over the levels for intervention and satisfactory control which would be agreeable to all partners, and 18 months elapsed.

Dr E offered the solution whereby each partner could indicate an acceptable range on each patient's hypertension card to guide the nurse. The other partners had not got as many hypertensives as the group member and so had less need or inclination to delegate their control to the practice nurse. The group member pioneered this for her own patients and when the practice set up a hypertension health promotion clinic, this was the style they used. In the end the group member's unilateral action served as a pilot for the practice.

Discussion points:

1 If a meeting gives one of its members a mandate, it must support that member. This partner should have been offered help earlier.
2 Leading from the front. One solution is to take a mandate and introduce change unilaterally. This is risky, but less so when the general views of the group are known. It can still undermine the person with the given mandate.

Every mandate carries accountability, and this should be clearly defined and understood. A time-scale for reporting back to the main group with clear criteria for success and failure are essential components of a workable mandate. These should be acceptable to the person who accepts the mandate. Judgements should be reserved until the review time unless disaster strikes.

However, if a mandate is demonstrably not being exercised effectively or if the mandate holder wishes to relinquish the mandate, the group must act to remove or transfer the mandate. The only way that a mandate failure can be consistently recognized is if, when the practice minutes record the original mandate, the time-scale is clearly defined and the topic returns to the practice agenda when the time limit expires.

CASE STUDY 13

In the winter before the new contract, Dr A's practice began to make preparations. One partner had been nominated as having executive responsibility for supervising the practice administrator and the practice nurses. Although he had protected time for these responsibilities his time was increasingly taken up with discussions with the practice administrator concerning the new contract changes so that the practices nurses were getting minimal supervision.

When the nurses needed help in preparing protocols for the new health promotion clinics, they approached a second partner. This partner approached the original partner and tactfully floated the idea that the responsibility for supervising the nurses could be transferred, but nothing materialized.

At a later meeting the original partner presented his problem of feeling over-committed in preparing for the new contract, and he appealed for help. The second partner re-introduced the idea of a transfer of responsibility for the practice nurses, and this was readily accepted.

Discussion points:

1 Transfer of the mandate.
2 Self-esteem. It is easier to accept a change if it does not imply failure – in this case in supervising the nurses adequately.

Clarifying current resources

Every practice has finite resources of time, money and energy. It is necessary therefore, when seeking a defined mandate, to offer the practice a cost-benefit analysis. On one side of the equation you will put the costs – time, money, energy – and on the other the anticipated benefits – time, money, quality of care, reputation. Only if the benefits clearly outweigh the costs will you want to seek a mandate, and the group want to give one.

For small changes the benefits might be so obvious compared to the resource costs that a formal analysis will be unnecessary, but every mandate giver will have the right (and responsibility) to satisfy him or herself concerning the balance of benefit.

There are two other important, closely related, costs to consider:

1 Will precious enthusiasm be used which could have been more useful or cost-effective elsewhere?

A practice and a member of a practice has only so much energy to put into development. You have to be careful that a proposed change will not detract from another change, perhaps one that is already in progress, or that the changes underway will detract from this proposed change. Try not to overload the system.

2 Will a better opportunity be lost because of this change?

A particular change is often chosen at the expense of another. If this is explicit, then a rational choice is made in terms of priority. If, however, the proposed change is seen in isolation, it may, on the surface, appear attractive. Only when it is compared to other possible changes does the case for delay become obvious. If you ignore this fact, then your carefully constructed mandate can evaporate when it becomes apparent which other opportunity cannot be taken up because of your change.

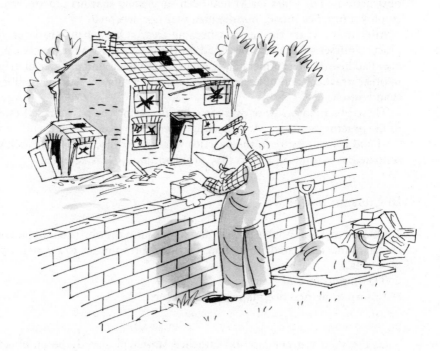

Identifying obstructions and planning to avoid them

A mandate is given by those with power, which in primary care means either the practice meeting or a primary health care team meeting. Tasks can be delegated, but the ultimate responsibility cannot. A practice manager might delegate the staff rota to a senior receptionist, but in a practice meeting it is the practice manager who will be accountable for problems with it.

Once a mandate has been given, it needs to be executed, and this usually involves people who were not party to the giving of the mandate. Before going ahead it is a good idea to reflect on the problems ahead (the potential obstructions) and how to minimize them.

Trying to introduce change without the co-operation of the people affected will never work. Their active help will make a valuable contribution to success.

CASE STUDY 14

In introducing new ideas, a team member needs to be fully aware of the obstructions. For years Dr M had been suggesting that his practice should employ a practice nurse, but the idea was not accepted.

After many years the reasons became clear. One partner believed that practice nurses generated work-load for the doctors. Also the practice manager had heard of resentment between practice nurses and practice managers in other practices and he resented the fact that a nurse would be paid more than himself.

These obstructions were overcome by increasing the pay and self-esteem of the practice manager. At a meeting when the perceived increasing work-load and time pressure in the practice were under discussion, the idea was refloated as a solution to this new problem, and it was accepted.

Discussion points:

1 One partner was unable to 'sell' the change until the obstructions had been revealed and addressed by making the idea the solution to other people's problems.
2 The importance of timing.
3 Ensuring the practice manager feels secure.

Ideally your partnership and attached staff will already be an effective work force but there are many contributing factors to such a happy state. Creating a constructive atmosphere includes:

1 Caring about people, and getting them to care about their work.
  After absence ask 'How are you? What was wrong? How we *missed* you!'
  For example, when a receptionist returns to work after a day's illness. The doctor says his usual 'how are you today?' to which she replies 'much better thank you. I am glad to be back'. 'I didn't know that you'd been off,' the doctor says before he realizes the significance.

2 Setting high standards.
   Be seen to be honest, fair, enthusiastic. Avoid promises you cannot keep.
   Let staff know how they are doing and what is required of them.
   Recognize effort and achievement. Praise good performance. Give
   constructive criticism as required. Help people to develop their personal
   abilities. Discourage cynicism, apathy and poor performance.
3 Encouraging people to tackle their work-related problems.
   Concentrate on solutions rather than problems. Help people to live with
   insoluble problems, support rather than sympathize to avoid causing
   inadequacy.
4 Keeping them informed of matters affecting them.
   Explain reasons for rules and procedures. Explain how people fit in and
   the importance of each individual contribution.
5 Dealing with grievances promptly, listening carefully.
   When a change is mooted, bear in mind possible reactions from your staff.
   If you fail to anticipate a problem, move quickly to identify the grievance,
   to explain and to mitigate the problem.

Remember that to the employees a decision at a management (e.g.
practice) meeting is an externally imposed change and it needs handling in
that light. Reactions to change may include anxiety, feeling threatened,
frustration, aggression, regression by sulking, assuming less responsibility
and even withdrawal by ignoring it, non co-operation or resigning.

The crucial aim in introducing a change is to ensure that those involved see
the purpose of the change and in particular how they will benefit personally.

Exercise 13

List the feelings and reactions you experienced when you first read the
1990 Contract.

Reflect on how many of those feelings and reactions are mirrored in the
practice staff after practice meetings.

The leadership of change can vary from authoritarian to extremely
relaxed, but is likely to be more effective when somewhere in between. Staff
left with a problem and told to solve it are likely to flounder so managers
must ensure that they give some guidance, such as the definition of the
problem and even some general directions for solution. By leaving the staff
quite a lot of freedom the manager will benefit from their early involvement
with the project. The more they feel it is their project, the more likely they
are to ensure it succeeds (sharing ownership). They are also often nearer the
ground and so see solutions more clearly. As always, use opportunities.

An employee or patient's complaint may illustrate the value of making the change. Of course much of what applies to the employed staff, applies equally to the partnership, as is illustrated in this case study.

CASE STUDY 15

Dr L had to confront the fact that her partnership was going through a very difficult time. All the partners seemed to be indulging in negative, obstructive and destructive behaviour patterns.

She called a practice meeting for which there was only one item: the partnership's relationships. After an open discussion they agreed to draw up lists of their own needs, specifically concentrating on what they wanted to get out of practice life. At the next meeting they compared notes, recording their feelings on a flip chart.

At subsequent meetings they addressed their communication systems, the responsibilities within the practice and operational difficulties. Although problems continued to occur, there was a better atmosphere of mutual understanding.

At a later date the partners had another 'squall' when communication lapsed due to holidays, and tensions built up. Based on the insights gained originally, this time they committed themselves to fortnightly meetings alternating between the surgery and the pub to ensure an informal setting. This allowed feelings to emerge before they got out of hand.

Discussion points:

1 A breakdown in relationships. Although this time it was within the partnership, the same could apply to relations with employed staff.
2 The methods for coping with major relationship stresses, including the technique of making things overt.
3 The confidence required to achieve this process. Often a confrontational approach to relationship breakdown can make people defensive. It requires mutual trust and consideration of feelings.
4 The short term gains and the difficulty in maintaining them long term. *Staff relationships need to be worked at hard and continuously to avoid such crises.*

Most changes in primary care are internal, but some have wide ramifications. A change in surgery times affects both the patients and, through terms of service, the FHSA. It is necessary therefore to look at each proposed change and reflect on its implications outside the practice. If you decide that people and organizations beyond the practice team are affected, then you must decide the extent and the necessity of involving them in the process of change.

It may be helpful to set out the obstructions in writing in order to clarify them. For example, a practice decides to start a cervical cytology campaign. The practice manager might identify the obstructions on a chart (*see* Table 1). Alternatively, the practice manager may use a blank chart and get the other staff to help identify the possible obstructions. This also has the advantage of leading to the early involvement and motivation of the staff.

Studying Table 1, and particularly the column 'how to minimize obstructions', makes it clear that definition of the current position is a vital first step. This is largely done by talking to all those involved. A blank copy of this table appears at the end of the chapter and can be used in your practice.

Table 1. An analysis of possible obstructions in a cervical cytology programme

	Obstructions	How to minimize obstructions
INTERNAL		
People (doctors, administrative, nursing)	time to take smears	look at rotas estimate time needed
Personal resources	misjudge initial commitment not all see need for it 'It threatens me'	talk to individuals reformulate the change create the right atmosphere
Numbers	resignation illness pregnancy holidays	check out with all involved
Time	too busy with acute work preoccupation with smears will put pressure on other work	
Equipment	computer breakdown question of sterility other demands on space	check equipment is adequate check priorities
Instruments	only just enough speculae	
Room	consulting rooms free, even if surgeries over-run?	
Finance	prepared to spend money if need arises? How much?	

Patients	high default rate due to holidays,
	  clinic time, previous unrecorded
	  smear etc.
		pilot project

EXTERNAL	Lab may refuse to take more slides because of backlog	check with the lab

CASE STUDY 16

Imposed change is most likely to encounter obstructions, especially when it is considered threatening. Dr R became involved in a DHA issue, where the resistance to change was one way of expressing underlying fears.

The DHA had decided, with widespread support from all paramedics, that a local long-stay unit should be closed but the consultant in charge was refusing to discuss a timetable. Since it was felt that a clinician might be best able to help this situation, Dr R, a local GP, was recruited by the unit manager to visit the consultant.

It quickly became clear that the consultant saw his job being contracted and that his specialty itself was under threat. After a long period of being harangued, Dr R discussed with him his fears and emphasized the clinical importance of a good discharge assessment and written summary when the long-stay patients were discharged. He reported to the unit manager in very pessimistic tones.

To everybody's surprise the first patients began to be discharged soon after and the consultant set a deadline for the unit's closure.

Discussion points:

1 The need to appreciate and value people and their fears. Often the obstructions derive from feelings – the consultant felt threatened by this imposed change.

2 Attitudes often change after sessions rather than during them.

3 Often an opportunity to express anger is very therapeutic. The consultant evidently felt that his opinion and feelings had been valued.

CASE STUDY 17

When the new contract was published, Dr A's practice went through the predictable initial reactions of anger and disillusionment. But the partners soon took an open decision to manage their way out of the problem and thereby to maximize the opportunities while reducing the drawbacks.

Copies of the contract were circulated to all the senior staff and a meeting was held to discuss their feelings. They discussed each area in turn, concentrating on defining the problems to be solved. This analysis went surprisingly well and the consensus was that all the problems were ones of workload and each could be done by a nurse rather than a doctor. It all seemed so clear and obvious that the meeting went on to design an advertisement for a full time practice nurse and to draw up a first draft job description.

Three days later the practice fissured. The attached nurses, who had not been at the contract meeting, were fearful that the new appointment would affect their hours and might even lead to redundancy. A discussion with the nurse manager quelled these fears but they were only a cover for the fact that the attached staff were fearful of the contractual changes which they did not understand and of the way the decision had been taken without their involvement. Insensitivity to these issues delayed the appointment and caused unnecessary stress in the practice at a time when there were more important concerns.

Discussion points:

1 Obstructions may not be obvious. They may be outside the zone immediately affected by the change itself.
2 The dangers of proceeding too far too fast: do not leap from problem definition to solutions without wide discussion.
3 Make sure all relevant people are involved, informed and consulted.
4 When problems arise, discuss them openly.

Identifying and mobilizing helping factors

The greatest asset that an innovator can possess is goodwill. Once it is achieved it needs maturing and jealously guarding, and it should only be exploited with caution.

Other helping factors are:

- A shared understanding of the problem and the solution
- Shared goals inside and outside the management group
- A clear and explicit mandate from the management group
- Wide sharing of ownership
- A clearly greater benefit than cost
- An absence of substantial obstructions, particularly ones that involve divided loyalties
- Waiting until an opportunity arises – such as a problem to which your change is the solution

The keys to mobilizing helping factors are explanation and sharing of ownership. Take time to get these right. For the previous example of a cervical cytology campaign, a written analysis of helping factors might be constructed (*see* Table 2). Again, consider whether your staff themselves could be involved in the exercise of constructing this, leading to a sharing of ownership and increased understanding.

A blank copy of Table 2 appears at the end of this chapter.

Table 2. An analysis of possible helping factors in a cervical cytology programme

	Helping factors	How to mobilize helping factors
INTERNAL		
People		
doctors	increases income	clear statement of income after cost deduction
	doctors believe they are doing a good job	show potential for greater job satisfaction
clerical and nursing	understanding of purpose	training and quality circle
	perceive benefit to self and others	training and financial incentive
Personal resources		
Numbers		
Time		
Equipment	any time-saving equipment (e.g. new sterilizer)	
Instruments		
Room		
Finance		
Patients	appropriate time of day	monitor attendance rate questionnaire
	good wording of letter	try it out on some patients
	GP, staff give personal encouragement to patients at consultations	keep smears high on the agenda
EXTERNAL	DHA publicity	good timing of invitations

CASE STUDY 18

In Dr C's practice, appropriate timing and early involvement of the staff led to swift computerization. Whilst the merits of computerizing repeat prescribing had been accepted for some time, action was precipitated by the imminent ending of the 'low cost' computer options and the 1990 Contract.

The staff were involved at an early stage, with visits to other practices to see the two possible systems in action. There was a rapid appreciation of the possibilities of improved registration details, help with the practice report and call and recall.

The chart for identifying obstructions (Table 1) was used and discussed by the staff. It soon began to seem that it was the partners rather than the staff who were dragging their feet.

When the system was finally delivered, the data were entered, checked and put into use in record time. The doctors proved slow in cleaning problem lists and making decisions over specific recording policies, but the staff momentum carried them forward.

Discussion points:

1 Early active staff involvement. They became the prime motivators of the change.
2 Staff involvement in identifying obstructing and helping factors. Staff involvement helps to anticipate and minimize obstructions, and their enthusiasm can be a key helping factor.

One method widely used in industry is to establish a 'quality circle'. This is a group of people, quite likely to involve a broad mix of very different professional groupings who get together to discuss the quality of service the organization is providing and to identify the obstructions to higher quality. They approach this by looking at quality from a consumer's point of view.

A quality circle in primary care might be organized by the pratice manager and include a doctor, a nurse, a receptionist and a cleaner. The composition would be determined by local circumstances but it should represent a wide spread of practice employees and might include a patient representative nominated from a Patient Participation Group.

Such a quality circle would then set out to identify the main problems in the practice and their causes. This analysis, along with suggestions for solutions, could then be put to the practice meeting.

The author's know of no practice which uses quality circles and we have not introduced them to our practices. We do however see enormous potential in the idea and will watch developments in this area with considerable interest.

Coping with imposed change

Not all imposed change is unwelcome. A pay rise well above the inflation rate creates pleasant problems – mainly how to spend it. However, most externally imposed changes, and certainly those that absorb most time and effort, are unwelcome.

In Chapter 2 six roles in change were identified. Three of these were essentially negative – consuming, obstructing and ignoring. These are the prime roles adopted in response to imposed change.

There are however some positive roles, and whenever possible these should be adopted:

1 Predict it, and plan for it.
   Often it is possible to anticipate changes that are unattractive but inevitable and plan to minimize their effect.
2 Create opportunities for favourable change.
   In the depths of every imposed change, however unwelcome, is an opportunity. It may be difficult to find, but once found it can help the process of adjustment.

Imposed change can come from many sources both inside the practice (internal imposed change), and from outside (external imposed change):

Imposed change	Source	Example
Internal	A taken mandate	The senior partner reorganizes the duty rota
	A management group	Decisions at a practice meeting are imposed on the staff
External	A taken mandate	The community nursing officer withdraws a district nurse
	A management group	The government issues a new GP contract

It is instructive to consider your own reaction to the 1990 Contract (Exercise 13), and the profession's reaction. Despite the profession having repeatedly requested changes to the old contract, when the new one was published most GPs reacted angrily.

Exercise 14

Consider again the reactions and feelings in response to the 1990 Contract that you recorded in Exercise 13. Consider also the responses within your co-workers and the profession at large. Try to categorize the stage of bereavement (*see* below) that your practice, and you personally, have reached in response to this imposed change.

Some doctors displayed another reaction. They reluctantly accepted that the change was coming and began to plan ahead to maximize the benefit from it. The best examples of this were the practices that made a cervical cytology action plan aiming to reach the new targets by the date the contract was due to be implemented, and optimizing item of service payments before they were withdrawn.

It is important to identify the type of reaction that is exhibited in response to undesirable imposed change, indeed to any unpleasant change – the bereavement reaction. Bereavement represents the worst imposed change, but the same reaction can be seen to behavioural change such as giving up smoking.

The bereavement reaction

- Denial
- External anger
- Internal anger
- Apathy/depression
- Acceptance

Not all these phases will be seen with every change, but all were observed in the response to the 1990 Contract. In bereavement the doctor will respond with empathy, listening, explanation and counselling. These are exactly the skills required when helping others to come to terms with imposed change, and an awareness of the process may help you and your practice to adjust as effectively as possible.

Examples of this abound but the following two episodes serve to demonstrate how negative reactions to imposed change such as anger, annoyance, and helplessness can easily spoil opportunities. In the first case it was only when the feelings were absorbed and time for reflection had occurred that the situation was accepted as an opportunity.

CASE STUDY 19

Imposed change often causes disproportionate stress. Dr N's practice was faced with cuts in community services which meant the withdrawal of the district nurse from treatment room sessions. The practice was not involved in the decision but was confronted with a 'fait accompli'.

The practice expressed its anger to the nurse manager who responded by offering to fund a few hours of a practice nurse if the practice employed one. The practice reluctantly accepted this offer, and on reflection later the group member realized that it was a good offer which would lead to the practice employing a nurse at last. Some good would come after all.

Discussion points:

1 Reaction to imposed change.
2 Some unexpected good can often come from a change, even an imposed one. In this case, the change resulted in increased managerial control of nursing services in the practice.

In the next case study the Pyrrhic victory may have been unnecessary if an understanding of the situation from the Health Authority side, and a consideration of the possible outcomes of their line of action had been carefully established by the partners at the onset. This process might have suggested that alternative strategies should be examined.

CASE STUDY 20

The local DHA unilaterally announced that it was introducing neighbour-hood nursing to Dr S's practice. This meant that long standing on-call rotas and inter-practice sharing of community nurses would be disrupted. Furthermore, the practice was to be in a neighbourhood that looked neat on the map but which was bisected by a river with no bridges. The number of hours of health visiting would be reduced.

The practice decided to fight. It remorselessly pointed out the absurdity of the new proposals to anybody who would listen and after six months the decision was rescinded. However, this was to be a hollow victory. The staffing was still reduced and the on-call rotas were disadvantageous to the community staff in the practice concerned. Most importantly, the image of the practice in the eyes of the DHA had been seriously dented and previous good working relationships had been adversely affected.

Discussion points:

1 Imposed change and conflicts of interest. Loyalty to attached staff and the need to maintain services conflicted with the desire to maintain a good working relationship with the DHA.
2 Open fights lead to open wounds.

Learning points from Chapter 4

○ When accepting a mandate, ensure that you know how far you can take it before reporting back.
○ A clear understanding of the initial position is vital before you can introduce change.
○ Staff relationships have to be worked at hard and continously.
○ The crucial aims in introducing change are:
  ● to ensure that those involved see the purpose of the change
  ● to ensure that those involved see how they will benefit personally
○ When imposed change is coming, make it work for you.

An analysis of possible obstructions

Obstructions	How to minimize obstructions
INTERNAL	
People (doctors, administrative, nursing)	
Personal resources	
Numbers	
Time	
Equipment	
Instruments	
Room	
Finance	
Patients	
EXTERNAL	

An analysis of possible helping factors

	Helping factors	How to mobilize helping factors
INTERNAL		
People doctors		
clerical and nursing		
Personal resources		
Numbers		
Time		
Equipment		
Instruments		
Room		
Finance		
Patients		
EXTERNAL		

5 Organizing the Process of Change – How Are You Going to Get There? (Part Two)

Contents of this chapter

Introduction

The last chapter examined the controls needed for managing change. This chapter looks at the organization required.

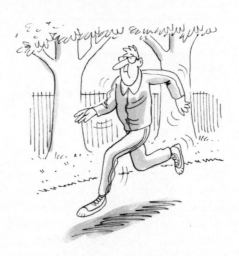

This is partly down to sensible practice administration. Meetings should have agendas, minutes and chairmen; staff should be properly appointed and tasks should be correctly delegated. Without this infrastructure, the process of change will get lost in the complexities of everyday general practice.

Selecting, appointing and supervising

Selecting

Before setting out to appoint a new member of the team, you, and your key co-workers, need to be clear about the following:

1 The reason the appointment has become necessary
   If it is a new appointment, then the problem(s) that need to be solved should be understood, and the aims of the change should be clear (*see* Chapter 3). If it is a replacement appointment, then revisit the original aims and check that a replacement is really necessary. Rather than a replacement full-time partner, have you considered two part-time partners, or even a nurse practitioner?

2 The job description
   This needs to be a written document for two reasons: it allows the team to check and agree the content of the new post, and to suggest innovations, and the written description helps prospective applicants to evalue their suitability for the post.

3 A profile of the ideal appointee
   This should be an internal document, but one agreed among the team members. Many a selection process yields an unsatisfactory appointment because the practice has not shared its vision of the ideal candidate. For example, when selecting a practice manager one partner may have a vision of a middle-aged maternal type, another a young businesswoman who goes in for power dressing, and another a male clerk. Until these differences are discussed and resolved it is unlikely that a successful appointment can be made.

Appointing

When it comes to appointing, the team must be explicit about the mandate for making that appointment. It may decide that everybody must interview the prospective candidates for new partner, but it must still decide who will organize the interviews, circulate the curriculum vitae etc.

It is usually not considered necessary for all partners to attend interviews for a receptionist post, so the group gives a mandate to, say, one partner and the manager to do the interviewing, one of whom is appointed chairman. It must be clear, however, that those two have the job of appointing and that other partners cannot veto the appointment later. It is important, therefore, that the people who will work closely with the appointee are on the interviewing panel.

The appointments team should advertise appropriately in:

- The local paper
- An appropriate professional journal
- Verbally to colleagues and staff
- Through bureaucratic channels e.g. FHSA

During the interview the chairman must exercise the skills required (see later) to allow searching questions to be asked and to give enough time for the candidate to sell him or herself. Always treat the candidate with courtesy and respect, thanking them for the interview and giving them a date when the result of the interview will be known.

When a candidate has been chosen and has accepted, ensure that all the team members are made aware of the result.

Supervising

Every appointee (including new partners) should have a clearly defined supervisor to whom he or she can turn for advice. This person should construct an induction programme and should identify and meet the training needs of the new staff member.

Allow an induction period with supervision and decide on a review date. This will give the opportunity for the candidate's abilities to be assessed and give the candidate the opportunity to air any difficulties they may be having.

Exercise 15

Review the most recent appointment to your practice. Decide whether the following were explicit, and written down:

- The problem to be solved and the aims of the change
- The alternatives to this appointment
- The job description
- An internal description of the ideal applicant
- A mandate to organize, select and appoint
- An agreed period of assessment
- A supervisor

Managing meetings and achieving chairmanship skills

'The English way is a committee – we are born with a belief
in a large table, clean pens and 12 men with grey hair'

Walter Bagehot

Meetings for their own sake are a waste of time, but meetings are a prime tool in the management of change. They are firstly about communication – information is shared, opinions are expressed and attitudes are changed. They are also about management – defining problems, considering goals, choosing action and monitoring the effects.

CASE STUDY 21

A partner felt that there was ample opportunity to discuss problems informally, however Dr D did not, but did not force the issue.

Some time later the health visitor told Dr D how disappointed she was at his negative attitude to practice meetings. This mistaken impression had been gained because the doctors were seen to be agreeing. This prompted Dr D to call a meeting with the nurses and to present it to the partner as a 'fait accompli'.

The meeting was not successful. Dr D discovered that there was another important meeting and began by apologizing for the need to leave after half an hour. The other partner stood throughout since he had 'other things to do'. The health visitor left after 15 minutes for a dental appointment.

From this inauspicious start the practice has subsequently managed to establish regular meetings.

Discussion points:

1 Meetings have to address an agreed need. Initially the partner was not convinced of the need and so he was obstructive.
2 The need to prepare well for new initiatives and to avoid diary clashes. The first meeting was arranged as a pragmatic response to the situation, but was not well prepared.
3 'Failures' may turn out to be successes. The first disastrous meeting was followed by the idea being adopted.

Skills of a chairman

Most chairmen are elected by the group they chair, and therefore have a clear given mandate from that group. Chairmen appointed by a person or body from outside the group have a taken mandate and need to work at developing that into a given mandate. Once a given mandate is achieved, the chairman's task will be much easier as the members will feel a sense of responsibility and ownership in its success.

CASE STUDY 22

Dr G had unexpectedly become chairman of a local political group at the request of the senior members. Although she had been elected unanimously she felt that she had not been given a mandate from the whole group. For this reason the first two meetings had not gone to her satisfaction.

She now felt that time, her own increasing confidence, and a recognition of her position within the group had improved her position. She felt able to keep the meeting to the point and to steer it in the right direction. She had started to engender some enthusiasm among the committee members – something she regarded as an essential facet of chairmanship skills.

As her role model she followed the skills of the chairman of another committee she attended. This chairman always kept to time, was composed and exuded confidence, and always allowed everybody an opportunity to speak. He understood the agenda and processes of the committee and appeared to know what decisions the committee needed to take.

Discussion points:

1 Problems of starting as a chairman. You can never be certain of the extent to which you have widespread approval or to which you are a compromise choice. It may take time to establish your mandate.

2 Gaining the mandate to lead. Whichever way you come to chairmanship, a solid mandate to lead is maintained by good chairmanship skills and giving the group a shared sense of purpose.

3 Chairmanship skills. This role model is an appropriate one and the lessons were noted, learnt and applied by Dr G.

Exercise 16

Write down a list of those meetings that you attend where there is a clearly identified chairman.

Consider the chairmanship skills in the light of each of the chairmen.

Write down a list of those meetings that you attend where there is no chairman and where the group regulates itself.

Compare the size and 'modus operandi' of the chaired groups to the unchaired groups, and reflect on whether the selection of a chairman might facilitate the workings of the unchaired groups.

It is vital to prepare well before the meeting. Study the agenda and decide on the format of the meeting. Try to be sure of the purpose of every agenda item − is it for information, discussion, or decision?

CASE STUDY 23

Dr J discussed the chairmanship of his practice meetings. Another partner had chaired the meetings but the practice had difficulty in taking decisions. Discussion tended to wander, often because the purpose of the discussion was not clear. Participants at the meeting frequently moved on to the next item before a firm conclusion had been reached. The partners reacted in different but negative ways. One appeared to block progress (a silent partner as described in Chapter 4); another seemed to opt out and a third became agitated at the lack of progress.

Dr J suggested to the practice that he should chair the meetings. The previous chairman, when he had recovered from his surprise, decided that it was a good idea. The subsequent meetings had agendas with each item clearly marked as to why it was there ('for discussion', 'for decision', 'for information') with a brief description of what the issue was and why it had been included. The new chairman would summarize each discussion with a comment like: 'I wonder if the minute for this discussion should read . . .'. Subsequently the management of change within the practice improved noticeably.

Discussion points:

1 The position of the chairman in facilitating and blocking change. Never underestimate the influence of a chairman in aiding or debilitating the process of a meeting.
2 Agenda and minutes. Ensure that these are accurate and informative.

If there is a difficult issue coming up it may be appropriate to canvass the views of the group membership before the meeting and, where appropriate, lobby in advance of the meeting in order to arrive at decisions. Lobbying allows members to formulate their views and the chairman to 'read the mood of the meeting'. It can also be a way of the chairman furthering a cause he believes in without appearing partial in the meeting itself, but this should be used with caution. It can provoke a backlash, and a failure by a chairman on an issue reduces his or her standing.

If a chairman wishes to champion an idea, it is often necessary to surrender ownership of that idea by selling the idea to another group member (see Chapter 2). The chairman can then remain impartial while the idea gets a fair hearing.

CASE STUDY 24

Mrs H, a health services manager, called together a task force of local 'experts' with a particular remit. She gave the full body a briefing and encouraged the members to give their views. At the end of this first meeting she specified the main job required and there was general agreement. She then appointed a sub-group to do this job and report back. The unusual aspect was that she did not put herself in this group; she appointed as group leader someone whom she had met that morning for the first time and gave the group total autonomy. All she asked was to see the documentation as it evolved.

The second example also concerns a 'hands off' chairman but of a different kind. This chairman was a man of clear thinking, incisive views and considerable wisdom. However, on becoming chairman he briefly introduced subjects and let the committee members debate at length. The chairman would then summarize, but the decision would by that time have become apparent. This meant that the chairman's views were not influencing the decisions and this made many group members uncomfortable. The first change came when that chairman took to briefing some members on his views beforehand so that they could be represented. This put those members in an awkward position, so the chairman started to give more directive introductions, making his view at least partially available, and eventually he joined in the debate if he deemed it appropriate.

Discussion points:

1 The extent to which chairmen should be involved in the debates in the body they chair. There are problems in being either too aloof or too involved.
2 Delegation. This involves trust and risk. A good chairman knows when to delegate.
3 Evolving skills. It takes time to know your group and to build up confidence; be prepared to alter your style if necessary.

Welcome the membership at the beginning of the meeting and work through the agenda systematically, allowing enough time for discussion. Summarize each point in the time allowed. Allocate an appropriate amount of time for each item on the agenda and keep to this (without sacrificing flexibility).

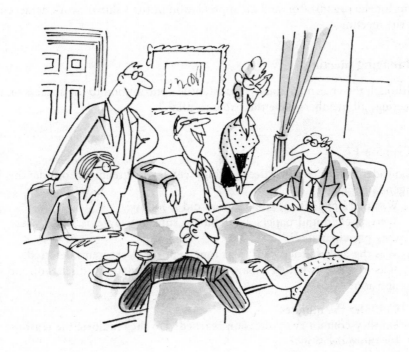

When decisions are reached, ensure that everybody understands what has been decided. Summarizing is a skill that GPs use frequently in their consultations. They summarize what the patient has told them to check that they have understood the patient correctly and they often summarize their opinion to be sure that the patient fully understands. Similarly a good chairman summarizes a discussion and the decisions arising from it to check that everybody has the same understanding of the meeting. Failure to summarize can waste the time given to a good debate. Make sure that accurate notes are made of decisions arrived at, and that these minutes are circulated before the next meeting.

Each decision for action requires a mandate and an individual or sub-group to take on that mandate. All too often a debate ends with an agreement on a course of action but nobody is clear who will be carrying out the decision. Set time intervals for reporting back and make sure that all this is recorded in the minutes.

At the end, briefly summarize the contents of the meeting, the actions decided and the persons responsible for their execution. Fix the date for the next meeting. Try to end a meeting on a positive note, engendering enthusiasm for the organizaton and an appreciation of the value of work achieved in the meeting.

Managing meetings

Although the chairman makes a substantial contribution to the success of a meeting, all members have their role to play.

Exercise 17

Consider the last two practice meetings which you attended. Consider the agenda paper:
  Was there one? If so, what format did it follow?
  Were background papers available on substantive items? If so, were they pre-circulated?
  Was the agenda followed? Was time kept to? Were items deferred?
  Was it clear whether items were for information, discussion or decision?

Consider the minutes
Do they contain every decision reached? Do they indicate the reasons for those decisions?
Do they show what action was to result from those decisions, the nature of the mandate and where it lies, and the time-scale for reporting back?

Someone must act as a secretary to the meeting and should ensure that there is an agenda, which may follow this format:

1 Apologies for absence
2 Minutes of the previous meeting
3 Matters arising from the minutes (these are what the chairman and secretary have determined from the previous minutes)
4 Any other matters arising (this allows time for other members to raise any issues)
5 New items on the agenda

6 Correspondence
7 Any other business
8 Date and venue of the next meeting
9 Items for the next meeting
10 Action by

In addition each substantive item can be labelled according to the reason for its presence on the agenda (for information, for discussion, for decision).

It is important that one person introduces each topic to be discussed. Ideally, that person studies the topic before the next meeting and circulates a written summary so that the other group members can formulate ideas.

CASE STUDY 25

This case study illustrates the dangers of failing to keep accurate comprehensive minutes. Dr W reports on the following problem in his six partner practice.

During a practice meeting the practice manager reported in a routine manner that 'the staff uniforms are arriving soon'. A week later over coffee, one partner said: 'I didn't know that the staff were having more uniforms. I thought we made a once-only contribution towards uniforms last year'. The other partners present all agreed with this, but none had felt confident enough to raise this in the practice meeting.

The partners decided to consult the old practice minutes to see what they had actually decided one year before. The minutes of the relevant meeting only said: 'Expenditure on uniforms likely to be £800'.

One partner and the practice manager had thought that the contribution was to be annual. The other partners thought it was a once-only sum. The minutes were quite unhelpful.

Discussion points:

1 The minutes did not record the important aspects of the original decision.
2 The need to voice uncertainty, even if it is unfounded, rather than keep quiet.

Use of time

Always start on time and always agree a finishing time. A good chairman will facilitate a meeting finishing on time, but over-running cannot always be avoided. The group needs to take the most important items early so that they have adequate time and any items which can wait appear later on the agenda.

Atmosphere

This should be warm and conducive to the meeting – not too stuffy. If it is likely to be a long meeting, there ought to be a break for refreshments. Members may need time to absorb the major issues and decisions. It may be worth allowing approximately one week for ideas to be consolidated in the members' minds before the decisions are deemed to be ratified. This particularly applies to practice meetings when the partners would not require a special meeting to ratify, but have plenty of opportunity to voice reservations if they occur.

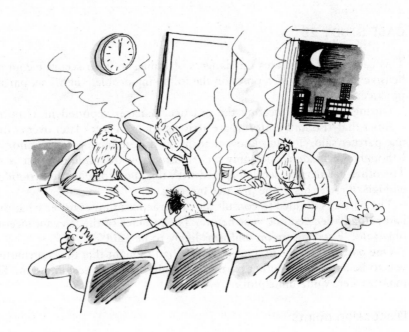

Time management

In Chapter 1 the importance of time in examining your personal position was discussed. Time is a finite commodity and you need to be able to make the best possible use of it – this demands time management.

Time management requires that you start with a firm awareness of your current time allocation and your ideal; the priority and stress of each time allocation and the task involved in each time allocation. You are then substantially on the road to deciding how to manage your time effectively.

Appointments

We all have appointments we need to keep. Louis XVI said that 'punctuality is the politeness of kings' but in a GP's case it is the lifeline to sanity.

There is no point in making appointments that you cannot keep. Running the patient appointment booking system at intervals that you never match; arranging to meet the district nurse in a patient's house unrealistically soon after surgery; or making business appointments with insufficient travel time between – all these just cause anger and frustration.

Whenever possible define your professional activities in 'blocks' and leave sufficient time to catch up between blocks. Within blocks minimize delays for you and the person with whom you have the appointment. If in doubt, audit it. Only when the true interval patients have to wait is clear will the problem become obvious. If patients are booked at an appropriate interval the surgery will finish at the same time with considerably less trouble. If a decent appointment interval is given and kept to, a patient with a complex problem will not object to returning for a second appointment. Another solution is to allow the patient to book the length of appointment that they think they require.

Travelling

Travelling time is, largely, wasted time. You should therefore examine all appointments that involve travelling. For the GP, are all the home visits necessary? Can some be delegated, or can some be avoided with a telephone call? Can some patients attend the surgery? Are home visit requests put through to a doctor or accepted by a receptionist? When setting out, plan your route carefully.

For a practice or nursing manager it might be necessary to consider if the person to be met could come to you; whether the meeting is strictly necessary; whether the issues are clear enough to avoid a further unnecessary meeting; and whether extra matters cannot be handled in a single meeting to avoid duplication.

Using the telephone

A pathology result, a request for a nurse to call, or simply a check on the response to medication can often be handled over the telephone by doctors. Do you have a time when you are freely available to be contacted on the telephone? If so, it can save many consultations and home visits.

Practice managers may find, for example, that the telephone is the best method to check how other practices handle rubella immunization. Telephone calls to three practices are quicker and likely to be more productive than a visit to one.

Organizing

In any day there are many occasions when you think 'I must remember so do so-and-so'. Often the thought is lost until it is too late. Try to either make a note or do it there and then.

If you keep an action list in your diary or personal organizer you will be able to regularly check on the things you need to do. The quicker you get them done the clearer you are about the reasons for doing them. Some substantial tasks require protected time. Identify when that time will be and be sure to address the task then.

Some tasks, such as dictating a referral letter, are accomplished quickly and are best done while the details are fresh in your mind. If a patient is late or does not appear, then catch up on such administration or consult your action list. There may well be a telephone call or a memorandum which can be fitted in.

Some tasks, however, seem to take on a dead weight, an active resistance all of their own. It is helpful to look at the reasons why this should be. Is it the boring nature of the task, a lack of confidence that you know how to handle it, or a time worry? If a task lingers, consider what is blocking you, and address that concern. All too often a deferred task becomes a millstone until it is finally accomplished – then it seems surprisingly small and quick.

Try to organize your working environment so that you handle things only once. Only handle the record envelope once per consultation; only handle correspondence once; only handle articles you read and want to keep once. Often personal systems for data handling let you down.

Establishing priorities

You need to learn to say no. You cannot do everything, therefore you need to identify those activities which are of greater importance – your priorities. When accepting tasks, have a clear idea of your goals in doing so and the time-scale involved. Just as groups have limited stamina, so do you.

Long term plans

In Chapter 1 the necessity of understanding personal goals was discussed. These were seen in the immediate context of establishing the way in which you would view changes presented in the near future.

In Chapter 2 the goal grid was discussed and in that you identified the short, medium and long term goals to which you were aspiring. In doing so you constructed a long term plan.

It is often helpful to have a written idea of where you would like to be in five years time, updated every few years when the old plan can be considered.

Apart from helping you to identify the skills you will require to achieve your goals, it will help you to establish priorities for your time allocations for major tasks.

Recognize time wasting

Idle chat can be fun and can help to reinforce relationships. Uninvited visitors may turn out to be stimulating and worthwhile. Meetings that appear dull can cover a vital and interesting topic. A car journey can help to get an idea into perspective. However all these activities, and many more, conspire to disrupt time management. Each should be used in moderation, each should be evaluated.

Monitoring change

Changes, like children, cannot just be allowed to develop unsupervised. They need monitoring, facilitating, correcting and caring. A neglected change will not flourish.

For every change a mandate must be given for its monitoring. Usually this is given to the person or group with the mandate to introduce the change, but it may well be another. A partner might investigate repeat prescribing systems and win a mandate to introduce a repeat prescribing register. The mandate for monitoring the working of the register might, however, go to the receptionist who generates the repeat prescriptions or the practice manager. Such mandates should not be left implicit – they should be clearly specified by the group.

In monitoring a change the obvious starting point is the aims that preceded the change. Is the change addressing the aims, is it solving the problems? Many aims are, however, long term and intermediate monitoring points need to be constructed, usually with a specified time interval.

Using the example of the repeat prescribing register, it might be an aim to have all 3000 patients on repeat prescriptions on the register within a year. That requires 250 to be entered a month – a figure that can be monitored month by month. If another aim was the identification of non-compliance, the number of non-compliers identified each month can be recorded.

Only if change is closely monitored will problems be identified early and will the nature of those problems be clear. It would be frustrating if at the end of a year it was discovered that the prescriptions had been entered incorrectly.

Another reason for closely monitoring change is that often other changes depend on the successful implementation of a first change. Unless progress is monitored, it is difficult to anticipate when the next change should be brought in.

Delegation and team work

Delegation is an art. It is never an abdication of your responsibility. It is a way of using time efficiently and of using the skills of others in the work environment. Never do anything that someone else can do for you.

CASE STUDY 26

Dr G describes a discussion he had with his practice manager. It took place during the turmoil leading up to the introduction of the 1990 Contract and the practice manager expressed frustration in her role. Her skills were not fully exploited and the pace of change had exposed conflicts of interest, differences in workload and clinical practice, and problems of leadership within the partnership.

The practice manager saw herself as being an 'outsider' who would be in a good position to take on the leadership role, and this contention was supported by her previous ability to organize the staff and handle partners. She attended a course on the management of change and, after discussion among the partnership, she was given a limited right to take a higher management role, including being an independent arbiter whose word would hold sway when the partners could not reach unanimous agreement. One partner was identified as her supporter in this initiative.

Discussion points:

1 Delegation. It is always best to delegate to someone who wishes to take on the task and who has the required skills.

2 Use of resources. The practice manager perceived herself as having untapped skills – no practice can afford not to use its human resources to their limit. This proposal offers an opportunity to exploit the practice manager's skills and to increase her job satisfaction, while achieving more objective, balanced management in the practice.

3 There is a choice between having the practice manager's role closely defined, which gives tight control, and allowing room for innovation and increasing effectiveness through self management which is the 'high risk, high gain' option. This latter course requires constant renewal of the mandate.

Delegation should be a positive act, undertaken in an informed manner. It is not a dumping exercise. The person receiving the delegated task should have it clearly explained and should, whenever possible, share in the ownership by determining how the task is to be done in practice. The delegation needs to be overt and the person to whom delegation occurs needs to know where the true mandate lies (the line of responsibility and accountability).

CASE STUDY 27

When the practice of Dr M accepted the need for new premises, it also acknowledged the time pressures on every partner. As a solution, they decided to develop a new surgery on a 'green field' site and to appoint a professional agent to act on their behalf in the purchasing, financing, design and building supervision. A partner was not given the task of supervising the agent who was left to his own devices.

This delegation meant that the project lost its initial momentum and this was complicated by one of the agent's companies going into liquidation. The partnership invoked a clause in the contract that allowed them to withdraw. This resulted in litigation which they eventually won. The delegation to the agent cost the practice over a year's delay and considerable anxiety.

Discussion points:

1 Delegation not abdication. As a management group, the practice meeting should never hand over a task to anybody and 'leave them to their own devices'.
2 Acknowledge mistakes and rectify them as soon as possible.
3 Delegation outside the practice. By all means use the skills of outside professions but be explicit about your requirements and supervise adequately.

Delegation works best if the delegation is willingly accepted and to achieve this it is often necessary to generate some enthusiam for the task in hand. Certainly its place within the practice should be clear.

Lastly, it should be possible for the delegated task to be returned to the mandate holder if the task is beyond the skills or resources of the person to whom it was delegated.

The need for delegation and the system for delegation are illustrated in the following table, which deals with a practice that decides to set up a smear recall system. One partner is mandated by a practice meeting to proceed, and faces two choices:

How not to do it	How to do it efficiently
The mandate doctor checks all the records of all the patients who need a smear (a massive amount of work). The doctor writes the letters by hand, the receptionist makes the appointments, the doctor sees the patients, does the smear, clears up afterwards and sterilizes the instruments. He then labels the bottles and fills in the request form to send off to the laboratory.	The doctor aranges a meeting with the primary health care team which is to be involved in the smear recall initiative. The attenders include the practice manager, a receptionist who is concerned with the task, and the practice nurse. In addition to discussing the problem itself, they have an educational meeting on the value of doing smears, the rate of detection of premalignant disease and how many lives the practice is likely to save by running its own smear programme. As a result the team members feel that they have a role to play in preventing disease and are highly motivated to make the programme work efficiently. Policy decisions (i.e. who needs a smear and how often) are discussed by the team as well as the mechanics of how a recall system might be set up and monitored. The doctor then delegates the task to the practice manager who instructs the receptionist on how to set up the register. The receptionist, who now understands the task, suggests ways of improving the register. Once the programme is running, the receptionist fills in the request form, the slide and the claim form, leaving the nurse to carry out the clinical tasks of performing the examination and smear.

The system described in the right-hand column makes sense for two reasons:

1 It is highly cost effective.

Medical time is the most expensive and the doctor should use it for tasks that others are unable to do. It has been estimated that the gross income from one weekly health promotion clinic could buy about half a full time receptionist.

2 By delegating you are making a statement of trust in your staff.

Using the skills of staff members and giving properly delegated and monitored responsibility increases their job satisfaction and helps to motivate them.

Exercise 18

Take one representative person from each of the grades in your practice – this might be a partner, the manager, a practice nurse and a receptionist. Do a rough calculation of the cost per hour of each person's time (ignoring common overheads) both in total and to the practice (i.e. with the 70% reimbursement taken into account).

Calculate the cost of a one hour practice meeting.

Learning points from Chapter 5

○ Appointing new staff is not straightforward. A systematic approach will help to minimize the risk of an inappropriate appointment. Where you cannot decide objectively between two people, be guided by your feelings.

○ Delegation and supervision are vital tasks that require skill and time.

○ Meetings are a vital tool in the management of change.

○ Chairmanship skill is not innate – it needs to be studied and worked at. A good chairman, supported by good organization, can be a considerable help in ensuring a worthwhile outcome from a meeting.

○ Time pressures are universal, but setting priorities, discriminating and delegating can all help to control time.

○ Change cannot just be left to happen. It requires monitoring and supervision.

6 Completing Change – How Do You Know When You Have Arrived?

Contents of this chapter

Introduction

In reality change is never completed. A problem may be solved; the original aims of the change addressed; the change may be regarded by everybody as permanent. However, problems evolve, aims change, and expectations are refined. With time what seemed like a reasonable and elegant solution needs adapting or totally re-thinking. How many practices put hours of effort into efficient manual repeat prescribing systems only to decide to computerize?

There is, however, the risk that a change will fail to establish itself, or will be reversed by circumstances. This chapter examines these areas and suggests that an innovator's work is never done.

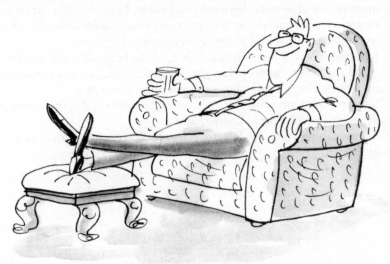

Assessing the endpoint

You can only assess a change if it is monitored. The endpoint is achieved when the monitoring indicates that the initial goal has been accomplished.

Matters are, however, seldom that simple. The initial goals move as a change comes into being. If an expanding practice decides to apply for a new partner, the initial goal may be to cover the increasing workload. However, while the partner is being appointed and introduced into the practice, all sorts of other problems may become important. The new partner might, for example, be seen as a solution to a problem with a clinical assistantship at the local hospital; or with cervical cytology; or computerization. If the change is only monitored and assessed in terms of the practice workload, then a success might be judged a failure, and vice versa. Now consider the new partner. Their goal might be just to belong to a friendly practice, but they might be very dissatisfied with the way the practice has handled their introduction.

It is clear therefore that the completion of change must be judged against both the initial targets and the floating targets that arise within the course of the change. Also, different people will have different criteria for assessing the change.

Your task, as a manager of change, is to keep this plethora of criteria under control, always explaining why some cannot be achieved and emphasizing those that can be, and are, achieved.

CASE STUDY 28

Dr P had wanted to change to ten minute appointments for a long time, but every time she raised the idea at practice meeting the other partners resisted—they feared the increased hours, felt that the time could be used better, and felt it was unnecessary.

Finally, she felt that something had to be done to help her sense of time pressure and, reluctantly, she decided unilaterally to start ten minute appointments but make her surgeries longer. She discussed it with the practice manager and the staff, but not the partners, and she monitored its implementation by gathering data on consultation numbers, note keeping, and preventive work. This monitoring showed that she was doing more case summaries in the record envelope, more immunizations, and keeping to better time. The staff reaction was very positive.

Two other partners quickly followed suit and another followed later.

Discussion points:

1 Demonstrating the value of change. In this example the change had to be sold inside rather than outside the practice, but the principle is the same. The monitoring persuaded the others of the value of change.
2 Leading from the front—a taken mandate. This is high risk but was successful in this case.
3 Blocking and helping factors. The benefit of reduction in time-stress was not appreciated and presented; the key people to make the new system work were fully informed and involved.

Unfreezing and refreezing

This heading embodies a useful concept. The status quo is a powerful entity and one that an innovator will use to institutionalize change. However, before change can occur there needs to be an acceptance of a need for change, any change. This process is called unfreezing.

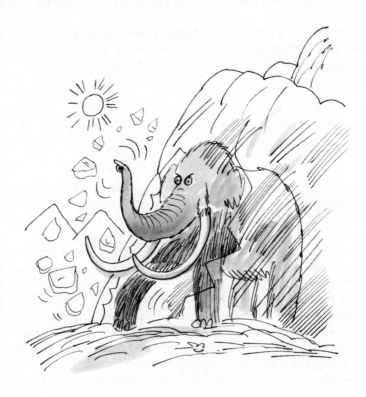

Unfreezing comes about in several ways:

1 *A shared problem.* Problems come to light in many ways, but it often takes a few small events or one big event to highlight problems sufficiently to make change possible.

A practice might, for example, have run its holidays on a 'first come, first served' basis. Only when the two younger partners have children at school, and therefore wish to adhere to the summer holidays, does a problem arise: they discover that the eldest partner who has no school-age children has reserved the middle weeks of the summer holiday. The younger partners feel angry, and the older partner feels aggrieved at being made to feel guilty for following the traditional system. There is a perception of a shared problem.

CASE STUDY 29

When he joined his practice Dr T found that cervical cytology was largely done by a Health Authority clinic and the uptake was low. The partners however did not perceive this as a problem. An audit showed the uptake to be 60% and the other partners felt vindicated—this was not bad—and no further action, including a call-recall system, was possible.

When the FHSA offered a computerized recall system the practice warily accepted and the uptake moved up to 90%. The FHSA system has however been a source of endless frustration and the practice has started to organize its own system, including its own smear clinic. Dr T is now seen to have been visionary and is treated with increased respect.

Discussion points:

1 Unfreezing. The offer of the FHSA system unfroze the situation, although waiting for this required patience.
2 Shared perception of problem. People's definition of a problem changed with time, in this case with the 1990 Contract.
3 The position of the idea generator. Even if it takes time for changes to be accepted, the original sponsor often finds his reputation enhanced within the practice—his ideas are listened to more closely next time.

---

2 *Change in circumstances.* Organizations, and particularly practices, evolve. This is another way of saying that change is endemic to one degree or another. One change creates problems that lead to other changes.

A practice may find its accommodation quite satisfactory until it decides to run prevention clinics. This requires a new practice nurse (and office accommodation for her) and somewhere to do the clinics so a treatment room becomes a necessity. Suddenly the topic of new premises which only a year ago was taboo becomes a high priority.

CASE STUDY 30

One of the problems of holding a responsible post is to identify a suitable successor. After five years Dr K felt that she was losing interest and had outgrown the job of being Secretary of a local political group. Two years previously a successor had been identified but Dr K had not relinquished any responsibility, nor had she attempted to train the new man in the tasks of the post. The nominated successor suddenly withdrew, and since there were no volunteers to take over, Dr K was left to soldier on.

A year later the chairman decided to retire and Dr K used this opportunity to discuss the senior posts with every member of the body. Not only did a new chairman emerge, but the retiring chairman offered to take over the secretaryship. As soon as this was agreed a member of the body volunteered to be deputy secretary.

Discussion points:

1 Unfreezing. The appointment of a new chairman made the difficult seem easy.
2 The problems of succession. Dr K failed to adequately nurture a successor. Remember that the longer you are in a job the easier it becomes, but the more difficult others perceive it to be.

3 *Imposed change*. Nothing can change the thinking of a group as dramatically as imposed change. Suddenly the unthinkable becomes thinkable. After the initial bereavement reaction (*see* Chapter 4), comes an acceptance and in this phase the opportunities lie. How many partners who have been fighting unsuccessfully for a practice nurse now find that in the light of the 1990 Contract the problem is to get the right appointment?

Exercise 19

Look at the changes that have been discussed and adopted in the practice as a result of the 1990 Contract.

Consider how much more difficult the adoption of these changes might have been without the externally imposed contract which has unfrozen the situation.

Consider your list of recent changes in Exercise 2. Consider how each came about, how the situation was unfrozen. Mark each according to the possibilities:

- Shared perception of a problem
- Changing circumstances
- Imposed change
- The skills of the innovator

CASE STUDY 31

A problem which reflected the way the practice meetings were run was reported by Dr Q. For 15 years his practice had used the district nurse to take blood samples from house-bound patients. As part of a work-load review the nurse manager decided that venepuncture for diagnostic purposes was not a district nurse task.

At a regular practice meeting, the district nurse told the doctors of this decision, but said that she would unofficially continue the old policy in the short term. The doctors were unhappy and a long dicussion ensued. A few weeks later one of the partners left a message asking the nurse to take a blood test and received back a message from the nurse saying that it was outside her duties. This caused considerable problems in this particular case since the delay with the message meant that the opportunity to process the blood had been lost.

A telephone call to the nurse manager clarified the situation and 'because it had been happening for so long' the nurse was given permission to restart taking blood samples. At the next practice meeting the whole saga was reviewed.

It transpired that the nurse was ambivalent about taking blood samples at home and that this was a hidden problem. It also became clear that each participant had a different recollection of the discussion at the first meeting. The nurse thought she had made the new ruling clear, two doctors could not remember, one thought the ruling was to stand, and another thought the district nurse had agreed to go back to the nurse manager to disagree with the new ruling. The district nurse felt let down by everybody.

The practice reviewed the whole situation concluding with a new arrangement that was agreeable to the district nurse, her manager and the GPs.

Discussion points:

1 The practice would not have considered this issue if imposed change had not made change obligatory.
2 Poor management process. The meetings are evidently poorly organized without clear minutes. This led to multiple misunderstandings and understandable hurt feelings.

Unfreezing can come about through a variety of circumstances, but it can be created too. In Chapters 2 and 3 we examined creating an unfreezing through gaining a consensus on the need for change. This is done by being sensitive to your goals and the goals of others, clear problem definition which gains consensus, and adroit management of the change process (sharing ownership, gaining mandates, etc.)

Allowing change to settle in

After a change has been instituted it should be allowed to settle in. This is desirable to protect it for revision (especially reversal) and to allow a reasonable evaluation of its benefits and costs. If a change is obviously useful then there is less threat to its continuation.

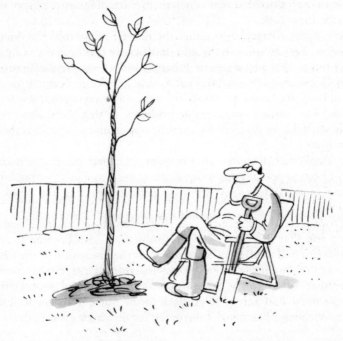

Some changes are more difficult to reverse than others. Once a new staff appointment is made, it is unusual for that person to be fired because the aims were not being achieved (although this may be the case if it is seen to be the fault of the appointee). Job descriptions can change, however, and the importance of the original task downgraded, or even neglected. All changes should be regarded as vulnerable. This is coped with in two ways:

Continued monitoring and supervision

It must be emphasized that you should not neglect change. Continue to cherish it by watching the process, detecting and correcting deviations early and maintaining the original enthusiasm.

Refreezing the situation

This is a natural tendency in any organization. Once a change has been absorbed it becomes part of the culture, part of the status quo. It can however be encouraged by demonstrating the success of the change (evidence produced by the monitoring), openly expressing satisfaction with progress, and discussing the next phases that follow on from the change as if the change were now taken for granted.

Freezing, it can be seen, is like much of the management of change, a psychological sleight of hand. The group members must believe in a permanency of the change and be prepared to fight for its continuation. This requires a group pride in the achievement of the change and a sense of mutual ownership. If the change was managed well through its inception, adoption, introduction, and supervision then this stage will come about naturally.

Completion

While change is a continual process, individual changes can and should be completed. Often this occurs at an ill-defined time and is only recognized in retrospect. For the innovator it has considerable importance.

It is often necessary to fix a firm time at which the full evaluation will be made and this needs to cover:

1   *The aims.* Have you achieved exactly what you set out to do? Or more or less? If not, why not? Think about optimism/pessimism, unrealistic or poor strategies, inappropriate use of resources, etc. Did you alter the aims along the way? Was this sensible?

2 *Method*. Did we do it in the best way? Consider use of time, people, resources, money.

3 *Cost/benefits*. Has the change been unsuccessful/beneficial? What are the spin-offs? Was the original cost/benefit analysis accurate?

4 *Other effects*. The participants – work methods, teamwork, costs. Other people – Have they been considered? Are all effects beneficial? The system – Is it working? Has the change been accepted/institutionalized?

There are several reasons why such an analysis is of considerable importance:

Learning lessons

Seldom is a change introduced in exactly the way visualized at its adoption. Some alterations are due to circumstances (other changes, especially imposed ones, affect this change—you are overtaken by events), opportunities (a job applicant has special skills which alter the aims) or other developments (a different method of handling the problem is published, a new computer company starts up).

CASE STUDY 32

Dr F's practice experienced serious problems with conflicts between the midwife, the health visitor and, to an extent, the doctors. It appeared that the midwife had a problem with low self-esteem so she did not contribute to practice team meetings; she also prevented the health visitor from sharing in the parentcraft clinics.

Dr F decided to intervene by meeting the midwife and the health visitor separately and counselling them. Almost immediately the midwife went on sick leave. Dr F felt himself absorbing the health visitor's anger at being leant on to run all the parentcraft classes, especially having been denied recent experience in running them! This storm was weathered.

Shortly afterwards the midwife became pregnant and indicated that she would not return to work.

Discussion points:

1 Good solutions sometimes do not work. The counselling approach was not given a chance to work before sick leave led to the total breakdown in the situation. However, the breakdown solved the problem, if in a brutal way!
2 Personalities. Clashes between individuals can be intractable and insoluble. Sometimes starting afresh is the only solution.

However, many of the alterations to a process of change are avoidable if the original planning and thinking are improved. This is where the lessons can be learnt. Failure to analyse the problem correctly, to stipulate realistic aims, to set achievable time-scales, to gain consensus, shared ownership or mandates, to monitor efficiently—all these failures contain lessons.

Learning these lessons can be personal and painful, but poor change should not be hurriedly forgotten. It is essential to reflect on all the possible ways in which it could be done better next time.

Reputation

If you have a track record of successful change it is much easier to carry your colleagues with you on a subsequent change. Such a track record may rest on illusions—others often mistake success in introducing change for successful results from change. It is, however, results that count.

The more ownership is shared, the less credit you personally will get for the adoption of a change, so it may be necessary to rely on demonstrating your skill in the introduction, monitoring and completion of change. This requires you to gather information and to have clearly defined intervals for reporting back to the group. This gives you a chance to sell your skills.

There is nothing more damaging than a reputation for 'not delivering the goods'. If you are bad at completing change, acknowledge this and make sure the mandates for introducing and monitoring the change go to a person with the completing skills. You then have to hope that your role in consensus building is recognized.

Exercise 20

Now that you have examined all the skills required as a manager of change, score each of them according to your perception of your ability at those skills. Use a scale of 1 (marginal ability) to 5 (high ability).

Awareness of personal goals	Awareness of the goals of others
Defining the problem	Gaining a consensus on the problem
Sharing ownership	General mandates
Formulating aims	Refined mandates
Overcoming blocks	Mobilizing helping factors
Using resources	Monitoring
Delegation	Completion
Learning lessons	Helping others to learn

Secondary changes

While one change is being monitored, the necessity for further change often becomes clear. This might or might not have been foreseen at the original adoption, but it must be perceived and reacted to as the change comes to completion. The new computer system might now be working just as visualized, and on schedule, but the staff are finding it difficult to keep up to date with the data entry and they need extra shelving for the computer terminals. If these problems are ignored the very success of the original change is jeopardized.

Having introduced the original change, the situation for staffing levels and shelving is unfrozen. You can now go for further changes with a high chance of creating a consensus, but this requires that you monitor the computer introduction and can identify that the change is complete. Otherwise some group members may, quite correctly, characterize the problem as 'teething troubles'.

Helping others to learn from the change

Primary care is highly parochial and insular, and there is a belief that ideas are not transferable. In fact the reverse is true. There is a variety of common problems, and many of the solutions and the changes adopted are adaptable to other practices. There are two main problems:

Ownership

If a practice generates a solution, it will be highly motivated to make it work. It will sometimes stick to it against all the evidence that there are better solutions elsewhere. Your task as an innovator is to help the practice to claim ownership of other people's ideas whenever this is appropriate.

Competition

In the psychologically competitive atmosphere of primary care it is sometimes seen as a failure to accept an idea which has been espoused by another innovative practice, especially one in the same area. Your task is to strip the idea of its origins, presenting it in a neutral manner. If possible alter some peripheral details so that, although the core remains the same, your practice can claim some originality.

In contrast, you need to help other practices to adopt your innovations if they have been successful. In order to do this you must achieve three things:

Publicity

This word is not meant in a vulgar sense, but a literal one. You must help people to be aware of your development not in an assertive, arrogant, one-upmanship manner, but in a constructive, informative manner. You should welcome inquiries, responding honestly with the benefits and costs and avoiding evangelical salesmanship.

Some ideas are publicized through journals, local newsletters and meetings and through databases (e.g. Royal College of General Practitioners centrally or its faculties), as well as informally in conversation with members of other practices.

Share ownership

Be prepared to highlight alternative approaches or mistakes that can be avoided. This allows the recipient of the idea to make alterations and share in the ownership. Bite your tongue when others then claim your ideas as their own.

Humility

Try not to overstate the significance of the change, and try to emphasize the team work that was involved. This allows others to view the change in its correct context and to assess its true suitability for transfer to another practice. This breaks down the natural resistance that can come from innovators being seen as, in some way, superior.

Learning points from Chapter 6

○ Situations change, and the unthinkable becomes thinkable. This unfreezing needs to be recognized and exploited.
○ After introducing a successful change, bed it in as part of the system.
○ Assess the extent to which the change has been successful. If it is not totally successful, learn the lessons for next time.

7 Practice Management

Contents of this chapter

The practice management task
The attributes of a good manager
The person profile
The job description
Conclusion
Learning points

Introduction

The medical partners cannot abdicate their role in practice management. They are members of the board of directors which can delegate to an executive—who can be a medical partner, a lay person or a combination. Some tasks, such as negotiation with the Inland Revenue, can be delegated outside the practice. There are few partnerships where the partners are prepared to let a lay person take on the full executive role and allow themselves to be managed. In these practices the lay person is truly a 'practice manager'—otherwise the correct title is 'practice administrator', which indicates that the managerial responsibility still rests with the partners.

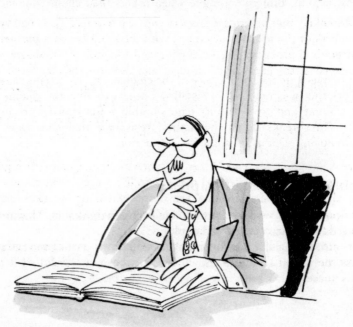

As expected, true practice managers are becoming more common. They are responsible for carrying out the decisions of the practice meeting, monitoring the progress of changes and reporting back. They instigate some policies but only implement them after the agreement of the practice meeting. This position is analogous to the managing director of a small company reporting back to the board of directors.

There is, however, one possible difference that needs to be borne in mind. Unlike many boards of directors, the partners are also key 'line-workers' in the practice and are the main shareholders. They therefore have a financial and emotional as well as cerebral involvement in decisions made by a practice manager. It is highly unlikely therefore that a practice manager will have sufficient delegated authority to influence dramatically the normal clinical process of the practice.

Some practice managers do, however, have skills in areas that the doctors do not, and in these areas they exercise most of their managerial control. In addition a good manager will become an indispensable source of advice and management skill so that in those areas which continue to preoccupy the partners the manager will hold considerable sway, including helping to manage the process of change.

This new role definition for the practice manager puts them on a different footing in the practice. Not only do their extra skills require a substantially higher level of remuneration, but they will probably become profit-sharing partners in the practice. This does not necessarily mean (although it might) that they will be on an identical footing to the medical partners, taking an equal share of the profits. It is much more likely that many current postholders will opt to have a fixed salary and an additional payment which is related to the profitability of the partnership.

It is also likely that practice managers with the required skills will become full members of the practice meetings, with an equal say to a partner.

Fund holding practices will be encouraged to employ a manager whose principle task is to supervise the budget and monitor the contracts. These managers will threaten the position and status of practice administrators. Real practice managers will however have the skills to supervise budget managers and will be in overall charge. The relationship would be similar to a managing director and a finance director—each have their own areas of expertise but one is accountable to the other.

There is however a great danger of specialist managers with high skill levels being introduced before the generalist practice managers have developed. This could unbalance the management of practices, pushing extra responsibility, against the trend, on to the partners and undermining the role of the practice administrators.

There are identifiable skills which the new practice managers require and these are detailed in this section. Also included is a job description and person profile.

The practice management task

Administration

It may seem perverse, having made a case for practice managers not administrators, to start a job description with administration. It is essential however that a practice manager has the administration of the practice under control before moving on to the other more complex areas.

This control will not normally be exercised directly. Most administration should be delegated. The practice manager, however, should be accountable for the quality of the administration and should sort out any problems that arise.

Administration involves overseeing the flow of paper—forms, claims, medical records, letters, messages, agendas and minutes, reports—that invade every practice. Meetings need to be organized and supervised, rotas need to be drawn up, filing must occur.

A good practice manager must be an efficient administrator, and the more transparent the administration, the better the manager. This is, however, only the beginning.

Information

Every practice does extensive information gathering, if only for its contractual annual report. The more progressive practices have realized that a key to successful management is good quality information and they have been concentrating on data for many years.

The information cycle is shown in Table 3. This cycle can be entered at any point, but is more effectively entered with either the identification of a new problem or initial data-gathering, which is usually designed to describe the situation in one area.

While this cycle offers a model for all data processing in a practice, it specifically addresses the problem of audit. A practice may start by looking, for example, at its care of patients with hypertension either because it is thought to be a problem or because it wishes to look to see if there is a problem. Either way an initial examination may involve pulling out the notes of 20 hypertensives and looking at how often they are seen, what the reviews consist of, what medication is used and what levels of hypertensive control are being achieved. This data is then transformed into information by being written up into a short report for the practice.

Table 3.   The information cycle

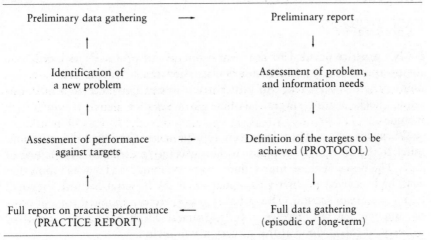

Preliminary data gathering   ⟶   Preliminary report

Identification of   Assessment of problem,
a new problem   and information needs

Assessment of performance   ⟶   Definition of the targets to be
against targets   achieved (PROTOCOL)

Full report on practice performance ⟵   Full data gathering
(PRACTICE REPORT)   (episodic or long-term)

From discussion on the report, a definition of the problem and a set of targets should emerge. These targets will consist of a series of statements which represent ideal care and a percentage beside each representing the achievement rate to be obtained. The practice might state that 'every hypertensive should be seen at least annually', but needs to realize that some hypertensives will choose not to attend, will be overseas, or may have left the practice. This statement will then have a level of attainment attached, for example 'to be achieved in 95% of cases'.

When a series of such statements are put together for one condition they are called a protocol. Protocols are by definition auditable, and the next stage is to set up continuous or regular auditing of the statements in the protocol. Some protocols, such as for childhood immunization, lend themselves to continuous monitoring, while others, such as hypertension, are best audited episodically—say every six months.

If the practice performance falls short of the standards set in the protocol there are two possible explanations, each with its own course of action. It may be that the practice is underperforming and that it needs to improve its care. This may require doctors to change or it may require the creation of management systems such as repeat prescribing, call and recall and compliance monitoring.

Alternatively the problem may be that the practice has set itself unrealistic targets in its protocol. Before the easy route is taken to reduce the targets to the level of performance shown in the audit, it is necessary to look carefully at those cases which have failed the criteria.

CASE STUDY 33

Dr N's practice decided to draw up a number of protocols including one for postnatal care. Without much discussion the following criterion was among the many agreed: 'All post-partum women will receive a full post-natal check at the surgery within ten weeks of delivery which will include . . . '.

When this was audited there were four patients who failed this criterion, much to the distress of the practice. This was interpreted as a clear failure of care. The notes of these four failures were examined and it was found that each had received postnatal examination at the hospital because they had had a caesarean section. The criterion was therefore changed to: 'All post-partum women will receive a full postnatal check within ten weeks of delivery. If this is done at the surgery it will include . . . '.

Discussion points:

1 Standard setting by group agreement.
2 Flexibility of protocol criteria provided the changes are clinically justifiable and can be defended.
3 The information cycle in action.

Information gathering is, as this book emphasizes, a necessary part of the management of any change—to define the present, to monitor the progress of change and to realize when the desired change has been achieved. The audit process is just one special example of the management of change—auditing is the management of change in the clinical environment.

In addition to the gathering of statistics, the practice manager needs to organize the collection of descriptions. A useful practice report (one that can be the foundation for the management of change for the following year) should describe the practice in numerical and verbal terms. To achieve the latter, the manager needs to get representatives of each group within the practice to describe the past year and the current problems on behalf of that group.

For example, reports might be written by one doctor, the practice manager, a receptionist, a practice nurse, an attached nurse, and any other staff that are intimately involed with the practice—physiotherapist, counsellor etc. These reports can tell the practice about those aspects that statistics cannot touch—morale, feelings and anticipated problems.

The definitive document for describing the practice is of course the practice report, but this is only a method, not an end in itself. From the practice report it is essential to develop a consensus on the problems of the practice and their priorities; the clinical and managerial targets and goals for the practice; and an agreed plan of action to achieve these goals. In other words the practice report (as opposed to the contractual annual report for the FHSA), is a vital tool in the management of change. A practice manager will make such a report the centrepiece of his or her strategy.

In addition to internal information, each practice requires an increasing amount of data about the external world. It requires information on the planned changes to the organization of the health service in good time to anticipate them. It requires social and epidemiological data, especially trends that might influence the clinical or organizational workload. Most of all, it needs information concerning the performance of other practices so that its standard setting in protocols can be compared.

All these information gathering tasks should rest with the practice manager, either to accomplish, or to delegate with supervision. If the power of the doctors in the practice rests in their clinical role, the power base of the practice manager is the information systems of the practice.

Planning

Based on the information gathered, a practice manager should undertake an annual review of the services and care of the practice, publishing it as the practice report (part of which will be the annual report now required by the FHSAs under the 1990 Contract). The practice report should state the overall aim of the practice and its specific objectives, present the current work both numerically and descriptively, and outline the practice's problems and achievements.

Using all the practice information and the practice report, the practice manager should be in a position to identify, after consultation with the doctors, staff and patients, the main areas for change and development, including their priority. Such a plan may of course be altered in discussion with the practice meeting before becoming policy, and requires regular review and updating.

From this practice plan, the practice manager should identify the resource requirements of the practice and prepare the practice's bid for resources to the FHSA in which the resources are justified in the context of current resource usage, the practice's identified problems, and the alternative applications for those resources. This will, in time, become a crucial annual document, the degree of success of which will exert a substantial influence on the development of the practice.

The management of change

Control of information is one facet of the management of change. Some unpleasant surprises cannot be anticipated but they can be alleviated. Most changes can however be anticipated, even planned, and can be controlled and managed. The practice manager requires skills in the following areas:

- defining problems and matching them to the goals and priorities of the practice and its members;
- obtaining agreement on change, including gaining the authority to lead it;
- setting targets and success and failure criteria;
- implementing the change including persuading the people affected, overcoming blocking factors and using helping factors, and monitoring its progress;
- completing the change and learning from its benefits and effects.

All these skills, and more, should be part of a practice manager's armoury. The practice may in turn delegate some tasks to others as a prime skill in the management of change is the art of delegation, with clear mandates, targets and feedback.

Financial

When one author joined his practice a decade ago he asked to see the accounts. Twelve used envelopes were produced, and on the back of each was a month's accounts! While things have moved on since then, practice accounts are still surprisingly crude in business terms.

Financial management can anticipate the troughs and peaks of income and expenditure, and can help to predict the effect of decisions that have financial implications. All too often a partnership chooses a computer or appoints a staff member with no clear idea of the implications for the financial well-being of the practice. Should they lease the computer or borrow the money? Will the extra staff member help to generate income and if so, how much can realistically be expected?

The advent of fund holding has created an awareness of the need for budgeting and resource control—a need which has been present in general practice for years. One spin off of this innovation is likely to be that the fund holding practices will gain the benefits of sound financial control of their business before conventional practices.

Personnel

The practice manager should have responsibility for all staffing matters. The practice's plan should include an assessment of staffing levels and requirements. The manager should be responsible for recruitment (although that does not preclude a medical partner being present at interviews for posts with patient contact). The manager should plan the training programme for individual staff members and the staff as a whole; should set personal performance targets for all staff members and monitor them; and finally should promote a positive climate among the staff.

This last item encompasses the need to communicate effectively with the staff, explaining developments and problems, and sorting out problems which the staff may have. If a staff problem relates to policy or if a problem proves intractable, then it should be taken to the practice meeting. One partner may be identified to give specific support in this area, but the first responsibility should rest with the practice manager.

Lastly, the practice manager is the conduit for views that the staff may hold. Of course these may be communicated informally to the partners, but the manager should funnel ideas, problems, comments and complaints through to the practice meeting so that the staff feel that their voice and opinion are heard.

Communication

Individuals in primary health care teams enjoy notoriously poor internal communication, while communication between practices, and between a practice and the health authorities is largely limited to contractual requirements and complaints. If a practice is to develop itself and its services this cannot continue to be the case.

No practitioner or practice works in isolation. Resources come from outside the practice and performance comes from within. Neither can be improved without co-operative effort built on common goals, and this requires communication. A good practice manager facilitates communication within the team, holding well-organized meetings with clear agendas, creating opportunites for informal communication, liaising with outside bodies and helping to spread an understanding of other groups' problems.

The attributes of a good manager

'A good manager gets 80% of the credit by doing
20% of the work'

A good practice manager should be able to accomplish all the above tasks and any others that are agreed with the practice. This requires various skills and qualities.

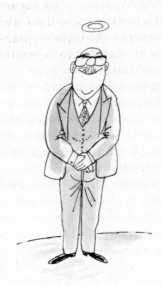

The first skill is in the management of change. All the techniques in this book need to be learnt and applied to the everyday working of the practice—usually without the practice members becoming aware. They might notice that things run more smoothly, but they need not necessarily know why. However, the manager needs to be fully aware of the process and to be prepared to change strategy if problems become evident.

The other skills are equally technical and may well be part of the armoury of an applicant for a practice manager's post. These are in personnel management, financial management and planning. The ability to organize information systems should be a priority skill.

The qualities required are those of a super-human. The prime requirement is for skills in interpersonal communication. If the manager can handle others with tact and discretion, humour and patience, and when necessary is prepared to surrender ownership or intellectual rights to others in order to achieve goals, then the battle is half won.

The manager also needs to be flexible, to welcome and find it challenging, and to be a persuasive advocate of change. This is not a plea for managers who opt mindlessly for change—any change—as the universal solution to problems, but for managers who are capable of evaluating situations critically and espousing necessary changes.

Perhaps the quality that is most required and is least often found is a sense of leadership. This is not a messianic standard-bearing fervour which drags the practice along behind, nor a passivity which permits total freedom for everybody to innovate in an unstructured manner.

The quality of leadership comes from gaining and maintaining a mandate to lead. This sort of mandate is given to those with clarity of idea who are able to create and maintain a consensus in the practice. This means that they work with, not in front of, the practice members, but their efficiency and ability inspire confidence and trust.

A good leader knows when to push an issue and when to let it rest, when to offer a lead from the front and when to give time for a consensus to mature. Such a leader is sensitive to the feelings and personal goals of others, but knows when compromise is a strengthening or a weakening manoeuvre.

Furthermore, a leader can take up ideas and sell them to a group, instilling a sense of mission or purpose in each practice member. This must be accomplished with a high level of self-awareness and humility, always alert to the need to accept fallibility and time for adjustment to the process of change.

If all this sounds too good to be true, it is. But there is no harm in identifying the ideal and then trying to achieve it. When seeking to appoint a practice manger rather than an administrator the doctors must accept that autonomy and responsibility must be delegated to a manager in proportion to that manager's skills with appropriate reporting lines, just as with a partner. They should then set out to find the candidate with the best skills and qualities that the practice can obtain and afford.

The person profile

When a practice decides to appoint a real practice manager, or to increase the skills of an existing practice administrator, it should examine the profile of the ideal person. This list is based on the previous discussion and can be used as a checklist to assess candidates and, perhaps more importantly, to create questions to be asked and aspects to be observed during the interview.

Attitudes

Must be committed to the success of the practice.
Must be interested in the efficient running of the practice.
Interest in maintaining good relationships within and outside the practice.

Commitment

Professional commitment.
Flexibility in hours of work.
Should mature outside professional involvement, but should keep it within acceptable limits.

Clarity

Ability to recognize important issues.
Ability to establish priorities.

Talent

Grasp a point quickly.
Think of a wide range of solutions to a problem.
High level of verbal and non-verbal communication skills.
Ability to express complex ideas simply.
Discretion.
Perseverance.
Accuracy in details.
Quick but flexible decision making.
Ability to delegate.
Ability to assert when necessary.

Flexibility

Tolerant of change.
Cope with stress (including that from practice staff, doctors and patients).
Tolerate frustrations.
Consistent stable personality.
Self-reliant and self-confident.
Good relations with staff, doctors and patients.

Interpersonal

Supportive.
Objective.
Tolerant.
Ability to understand other people's feelings.
Managerial experience.
Academic level.
Health.

The job description

Every appointee to a practice requires a job description, and with a practice
manager's post this is especially important. It is unreasonable to complain
that somebody has not lived up to your expectations if those expectations are
not clearly expressed in advance; equally it is unreasonable to expect a high
quality candidate to accept a job that is undefined except that it is surround-
ed by high hopes and vague expectations.

Although each practice should draw up its own job description, this draft may help by acting as a starting point. It is designed to cover the mission and tasks of a practice manager in today's working environment and does not include the possibility of being a voting, profit sharing practice partner.

Main purpose

To help the Primary Health Care Team (including the doctors) to deliver good quality health care to the practice list in a happy and progessive way.

To help to manage the changes in the practice so that the energy and resources of the practice are used most efficiently.

Achievement of these broad goals will require:

Personnel

Interviewing, appointing, supervision/overseeing, controlling, training and welfare of the staff, including instituting a career plan for individual staff member's development.

Instigating and implementing regular staff pay increases. Planning and organizing holiday and sickness cover.

Acting as personnel officer for staff and patients, ensuring enquiries and complaints are dealt with, investigated and reported.

Dealing with non-medical problems for GPs.

Undertaking disciplinary procedures as required.

Issuing and maintaining contracts of employment.

Finance

Controlling staff salaries, calculations, cheques and analysis book; calculation of ANC claims, completion and submission of all forms to the FHSA.

Submitting forms for salary reimbursement to the GPs.

Accounting for and maintaining petty cash.

Understanding and implementing the Statutory Sick Pay regulations.

Controlling the staff PAYE and Inland Revenue annual returns.

Being responsible for the partnership accounts, including routine negotiations with accountants and preparation of annual accounts to their requirements.

Offering advice to the partnership on financial control and budgeting.

Communication	Circulating information, organizing meetings, interviews, films, lectures and committee meetings. Ensuring that formal meetings are well prepared, with agendas, minutes and action lines. Liaising with the doctors, the FHSA and DHA staff. Facilitating the development of teamwork. Receiving and liaising with medical representatives.
Information	Setting up and maintaining appropriate information systems with the practice. Editing the annual report; facilitating the setting of group goals and the monitoring of their achievement. Developing the practice business plan and negotiating its acceptance with the FHSA; monitoring the practice's progress against the business plan and the FHSA's compliance. Maintaining the practice formulary. Organizing the managerial and clinical audits of the practice.
Doctors	Organizing the ordinary, holiday and sickness rotas to ensure adequate clinical cover. Arranging practice, managerial, educational and social meetings.
Office/ reception	Organizing and supervising reception and office procedures. Initiating new procedures to aid practice organization, streamlining methods, undertaking surveys, and delegation of workload.
Surgeries/ clinics	Allocating accommodation and ensuring smooth running of surgeries/clinics, including preparation of rooms and equipment, and adequate staff cover.
Visitors	Receiving visitors, organizing their visits.
Documentation	Documentation of statistics, staff records and forms. Ordering and controlling stores, equipment, medical supplies, furniture and fittings, stationery and maintaining inventory. Issuing guidelines for all new, improved or changed routines. Dealing with non-medical correspondence. Maintaining current records of all relevant information and instructions, minutes of meetings, and ensuring that appropriate action is taken.

Safety and security	Instituting/organizing safety procedures (fire) and investigating accidents on premises. Ensuring that staff are aware of security arrangements. Keeping accident book and other statutory duties.
Premises	Overall control and supervision of cleanliness, hygiene, appearance and routine maintenance of premises, and proper working conditions. Supervising all contract supplies and services.
Pension scheme	Controlling staff pension schemes, new applicants proposal forms, liaising with insurance broker and calculating correct salary reductions. Initiating and implementing pension increases, notification to and claim of reimbursement from the FHSA. Dealing with withdrawal of policy and amount claimed. Arranging alteration of direct debit for bank accounts.

These tasks are not exhaustive and the practice manager must be prepared to negotiate variations in the job description. Tasks that appear on this list will be the responsibility of the practice manager, who will be accountable for them to the medical partners through the practice meeting. The practice manager may however delegate any of these areas to other members of staff, provided such delegation is appropriate and supervised.

All these tasks will need to be undertaken with the co-operation and knowledge of the medical partners, and their execution will need to be sufficiently skilled to earn and maintain confidence in the practice manager's abilities.

Conclusion

Any person and any practice can manage change more efficiently. However, organization becomes increasingly important as the practice grows and the role of a true practice manager becomes central. Such a manager may be a medical partner, but it is more likely to be somebody employed specifically for the task. This section has explained the role, skills and qualities of such a practice manager.

Learning points from Chapter 7

○ Doctors have no god-given skill to manage; it is usually necessary for a practice to buy in these skills.
○ There is a clear difference between practice administrators and practice managers. Practices will be increasingly seeking the latter.
○ If a practice is clear about the type of person and the skills required, it is likely to make a more effective appointment.
○ A job description is particularly important for a senior post such as a practice manager.

Bibliography

Atkinson C J, (1989) Donning a manager's cap: will GPs be able to cope with the more managerial role dictated to them in the White Paper? *Health Service Journal.* 1218–9.

Beer M and Walton A E (1987) Organizational change and development. *Annual Review of Psychology.* **38**, 339–67.

Crouch A and Yetton P (1987) Management behaviour, leadership style and subordinate performance: an empirical extension of the Vroom-Yetton conflict rule. *Organizational Behaviour and Human Decision Processes.* **39**, 384–96.

Dobbs M F (1987) Organizational development interventions: a comparative study. *Dissertation Abstracts International.* **47**, 6116.

Eden D (1985) Team development: a true field experiment at three levels of rigor. *Journal of Applied Psychology.* **70**, 94–100.

Falk R (1983) *The business of management.* Penguin Books, London.

Fraucheux C, Amado G and Laurent A (1982) Organizational development and change. *Annual Review of Psychology.* **33**, 343–70.

Hastings C, Bixby P and Chaudhry-Lawton R (1986) *Superteams: a blueprint for organizational success.* Fontana, London.

Hunt J (1981) *Managing people at work.* Pan Books, London.

Pedler M and Boydell T (1986) *Managing yourself.* Fontana, London.

Plant R (1987) *Managing change and making it stick.* Fontana, London.

Pugh D S, Hickson D J and Hinings C R (1989) *Writers on organizations.* Penguin Books, London.

Sidney E, Brown M, and Argyll M (1984) *Skills with people: a guide for managers.* Century Hutchinson, London.

Williams R W (1986) Introduction of a management structure in group general practice. *Journal of Management in Medicine.* **1**, 158–66.

Index